MW00395700

"Elizabeth Frediani has done a brilliant job of writing a well-organized and easy-to-follow lesson plan for all to reach the important goal of spiritual self-care."
—Sandra Ingerman
Author of *How to Heal Toxic Thoughts* and *Medicine for the Earth: How to Transform Personal and Environmental Toxins.*

"Elizabeth Frediani has perfected a way to communicate practical and spiritually enriching exercises that are essential for anyone interested in living a holistic lifestyle. This profound coursework on mastering subtle energy makes the intangible parts of living clear and accessible."
—Joanne Saltzman
Founding Director of the School for Natural Cookery and author of *Amazing Grains, Romancing the Bean,* and *Intuitive Cooking.*

"*Where Body Meets Soul* teaches energetic practices to balance all the giving and doing in our lives. There is wisdom on every page of this book for those pursuing their personal truth and path to health and wholeness."
—Barbara Dahl, RN
Certified Healing Touch Instructor

"*Where Body Meets Soul* is a heartfelt and inspiring guide to working with subtle energies .... The readers who use this book as a manual for practice and spiritual development are sure to undergo a process of transformation that will leave them far more aware, balanced, and healed in body and soul."
—Robert Ullman, N.D.
Co-author with Judith Reichenberg, N.D. of *Ritalin-Free Kids, Prozac-Free, Rage-Free Kids, Homeopathic Self-Care,* and *Mystics, Masters, Saints, and Sages: Stories of Enlightenment.*

Where Body Meets Soul

Subtle Energy Healing Practices
for Physical and Spiritual Self-Care

Elizabeth Frediani

Singing Mountain
Publishing Alliance
2008

Published by
Singing Mountain Publishing Alliance
PO Box 1634
Langley, WA 98260

The exercises presented in this book are intended to expand your knowledge and practice of self-care, but should not be considered as a replacement for required medical or psychological care with a health professional.

Where Body Meets Soul:
Subtle Energy Healing Practices for Physical and Spiritual Self-Care

Library of Congress Control Number: 2008910904

ISBN: 978-0-615-22595-1

Cover photograph by Carl Andersen

To my early companions and invaluable guides –
Gary, Juli, and Dale

Acknowledgments

ONE OF THE CORE UNDERSTANDINGS of my heart – the truth that always awakens me to healing, gratitude, and grace – is that *life unfolds. I am unfolding.* And so, I see the journey of this book.

Karmic friends and soul partners, past and present, contribute to these pages, as they do to my own life. Dale Sachs and I went to British Columbia to seek sanctuary during the Viet Nam war. He has said that I saved his life. I say that he delivered me to mine, to my spiritual opening that could have only happened *there* in the mystic embrace of nature and solitude.

I am grateful for Gary Weidner, for our meeting at the perfect moment. His love, respectfulness, and his connection to the Earth led me further spiritually – and geographically – than I would have gone by myself. Deepest thanks to Juli Spencer, for listening and being present in the beginning.

A.T. Birmingham-Young is the editor and midwife of this book. Her talent and unwavering direction to *write true to my experience* sustained me through the long process of fulfilling my intention. I am grateful for our creative partnership and her gentle, restrained brilliance.

Clients, students, and trainees hold this book in guardianship. They have made their own commitment to the book's fulfillment by investing their time and focusing their healing efforts on these practices. I honor them and wholeheartedly thank them for the last twenty-eight years. Warmest thoughts and gratitude to

Peshali Yapa, Mark Rohde, and Yoshiko Iwakiri who re-ignited my interest in writing – and to Sadie Salim who enthusiastically added insightful, practical direction.

Where Body Meets Soul reflects much of the spiritual understanding I have gleaned through my long relationship with a community of Light Beings. To them I owe the inspiration of my work, my inner silence, and my absolute trust in the transformational process. Within the universal collective, we, the whole of humanity, are valued and aided. *Our work is to listen –* then live in a manner that expresses our individual gifts and serve according to our chosen commitments.

Rolling Thunder – in life and in the spirit world he keeps to his word to tend to what is needed. *I thank you for your love and support.* Sincerest thanks to Elmer Green, a dedicated spiritual pioneer and R.T.'s friend, who I have met through this book's emergence. He is an openhearted, delightful human being, who contributes much to many.

I greatly appreciate the creative input of my son, Sun Sachs, who was born in British Columbia and still carries the rhythm of that wilderness within him. I thank my friend, Carl Andersen, for his time, intention, and his intimate, powerful view of the forest for the cover. And, to Sandy Welch for seaming images, ideas, and linear details together – her patience and collaborative spirit have eased and enriched this creative process.

And last, I acknowledge my granddaughters, Lia and Fiona, who sparkle with exuberance and pure fire. *This book is from your grandmother, and it is a part of you.*

Contents

Preface

My passion for writing *Where Body Meets Soul* comes from knowing that each one of us can learn to nurture and protect our wholeness. And through this conscientious care of self we can increase our capacity to heal, to evolve, and to live authentically. I also recognize, as perhaps do you, that self-care dovetails with world-care. What we as individuals resolve, heal, and actualize contributes to a shift in the consciousness of us all. Our contribution to collective awareness can transform, illuminate, re-create. And now is a time for re-creation.

Subtle energy healing offers us a strong paradigm for transformation that advances both planetary and personal change. Through this modality we experience – rather than simply theorize – that *all is energy*. And, it is this reality, embraced by both mystics and scientists, that is re-writing the foundational premises of Western medicine, psychology, and spirituality. When applied in our own lives, subtle energy practice and methodology foster greater physical-spiritual integration, while opening many inroads to effective self-healing.

If you are currently challenged by a physical illness or particular life stress, this book will offer you numerous resources. Subtle energy practice is deeply integrative. It invites you, the practitioner, to cultivate wholeness. The body-mind-soul is a complete spectrum of energies – partly manifesting as physical, partly resonating at the subtlest realms of consciousness. All comprise self. Through subtle energy practice you will develop a cohesive connection to *your living energy*. And, it is this internal bond that ultimately restores, balances, and heals.

If you are a health care professional committed to expanding your understanding of subtle energy healing, the information presented here will support and guide you in this purpose. I wholeheartedly recommend you explore the exercises as a student first, however. Through experiencing their simplicity, as well as their depth and practical application, you will become a stronger resource for your clients and patients – and a more generous healer to yourself.

Spiritual practice is an integral part of subtle energy healing – and is, therefore, a core theme of this book and my work. We inhabit elegantly constructed and unified physical-energetic-spiritual bodies. Our ability to enter transcendent states of awareness, to develop unwavering compassion, and to maintain deep inner stillness and peace is natural to the body-mind-soul. Subtle energy practice uses the energy system as the path to these experiences. The heart center serves as the gateway.

As each of us nourishes and strengthens our whole being to reach soul-level integrity, we transmit a healing catalyst into the field of unified consciousness and help establish a greater depth of coherence on Earth.

May we all realize our potential as conduits for creative and conscious evolution —

Elizabeth Frediani
Whidbey Island
October 2008

Where Body
Meets Soul

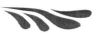

Introduction

YOUR BODY *DOES* MEET YOUR SOUL. They directly connect in your deep heart, in the energy center just above the base of your sternum. Here, near the core of your body, rests a point of interface between your physical being and your purely transcendent self. And to know this place – and be present in it – is to realize that you can always choose peace, compassion, and spiritual revitalization.

To find this place you do not need to clear your thoughts or *do* anything extraordinary. You need only learn to connect with your body in an informed way – understanding your subtle energy system, its attributes and design.

Seamlessly integrating physicality and spirit, your energy system is the living blueprint for the whole of you. Central to your body's health, it regulates your ability to receive, circulate, transmit, and conserve life force energy. As the mirror of your consciousness, it carries all the qualities and conditions of your thoughts, beliefs, and emotions. Your energy system also embodies your spiritual centers and, thus, facilitates the subtlest dimensions of your awareness.

This broad range of faculties and functions lends itself quite naturally to healing and self-care, since access to the energy system is easy and direct. Energy exercises, called *practices*, provide instruction and the guided steps. Using them you can learn to discern the causal factors of physical, mental, and emotional stress, balance and heal the body, initiate meditation, transform limiting behavior and beliefs, and experience greater spiritual connectedness. Developing in-depth energy skill simply requires practice and a shift in focus – a shift from the linear mind to a subtler, sensory connection with self.

My own recognition of subtle energy occurred over thirty years ago in the pristine wilderness of British Columbia. It happened gently and spontaneously through my living close to nature and the Earth. And although I had no points of reference for what I experienced then, I intuitively knew the value of it. I write this book after decades of teaching and witnessing the dynamic relationship between the subtle energy system and health, consciousness, spirituality, and selfhood.

Where Body Meets Soul, like the companion course that I have taught since 1984, presents an integrated learning process, which addresses your ongoing needs for self-healing, revitalization, and transformation, yet affords you much more. This material invites you to experience and affirm what you inherently know about your physical-spiritual being – *that you are sacred.* Fully honoring this truth is essential to heal *and* to live.

Meeting Light: My Personal Story

In August of 1972, my family and I moved to a home on one hundred acres at the foot of a mountain, named the Mountain of Many Voices – a place where First Nations people once thrived. Our land bordered no other home sites. Forest flanked us on three sides. At the rear of the house, the trees extended up the mountain to the clearing at an abandoned fire lookout station. Coyotes, cougar, pika, hawks, and ravens were our closest visible neighbors.

I came to love the land quickly. Interested in the variety of conifers that grew around us, I often explored the forest on trails tamped down by deer that I never actually saw. These winding paths led me up the steep mountain to places I would not have otherwise found – tucked away shelters, hidden by low-lying branches or outcroppings of rocks. Beds of flattened grasses held the impressions of deer that last rested there. From these tender homes I always carried back small treasures like stones, matted lichen, or pinecones to set in our rooms, so we would remember that we were now living on *their* land.

When autumn came and the days quickly shortened, I spent little time walking the forest. Instead I concentrated on readying our family for winter – canning the last tomatoes and purchasing bulk food from the local co-op. It was in those crisp evenings of early October that I began to hear distant singing stream down the mountain and lilt through the trees behind the house. The melodic voices of women and children came on nights that were exceptionally still and when the house was quiet. My young son was asleep; my husband was at work. I would step onto the porch to listen and to gaze into the stand of spruce just beyond the fence. I never once saw anyone, but often felt presences in the days that followed. On the forest path in certain clearings I would feel a palpable sensation of others standing close to me. There was a comfort in this, which I never questioned. I simply accepted it as I did the singing, and spoke of it to no one.

That same fall I had another new experience. One day as I sat to rest in the sunniest room of our house, the immense quiet of this land, which I had always perceived as merely an absence of noise, became subtly audible to me. As I listened, the *hum* of it drew my focus to the center of my head, then into the center of my body. I began to feel simultaneously awakened and relaxed. The interior core of my body felt remarkably fluid, and if I moved even slightly, streams of sensation would spiral around my spine. Each physical sound I heard – the rustling of fallen leaves, the cries of the hawks, the back door knocking from the wind – penetrated to the center of my body and filled me with an inexplicable vitality.

The first time I had this experience, I sat for only half an hour.

When I finished and began to prepare dinner, I felt an amazing sense of exhilaration that continued through the entire evening. After sitting one or two more times over the next week and feeling the same result, I decided to tell my husband. His response was definitive – "Oh, you are meditating." I resisted his explanation. I preferred the experience unnamed.

My exploration of silence and the inner world of my body heightened in 1973 after we moved north to a two-thousand-acre farm that sat at the west end of a long, narrow lake. Five hundred miles from populated areas, further into the welcoming solitude of nature, the hum did not require my sitting still to hear. It was loud enough to stop my conversation at the dinner table.

Soon after settling into the new house, I began a habit of taking afternoon walks. I walked, focused on the interior of my body, through the grove of golden poplar trees that bordered the lake's shore. One day I began to hear the sounds around me – the pulse of the trees, the voices of the loons, the whirring wings of the geese – as if they were the internal sounds of my own breaths. I immediately felt the familiar, deep calm and vitality fill me.

As I continued to walk, each step I took on the Earth felt like a movement that originated from somewhere beyond my body. While walking intentionally connected to this sensation, I experienced passing *from* the physical world. My eyes were open and I was still moving; yet, the scenery had changed. The physical world was gone. A shimmering sea of fluid light had taken its place. I do not know how much time passed before I realized that I could reverse my depth of focus and bring myself back to physicality. Upon my return, my words to myself were swift – "The world needs this."

When I first saw beyond the physical world, the light instantly informed and educated me. This new place was vital and vibrating but not at all foreign or frightening. I could see it with my eyes and feel it with my body. And, whenever I returned from it, a share of its reality came with me. In a completely instinctual way, I knew I belonged to both worlds, and both worlds belonged to each other.

Seeking and Finding Context

From that first autumn on the mountain to the moment I had a working knowledge of subtle energy took approximately ten years. Within days of first walking from the physical world, I began to see what I now know as energy fields – around most things and people. My new sight happened spontaneously and although I trusted the experience, I had no idea what was actually happening.

I soon felt compelled to study anything that seemed even remotely connected with what I *knew.* I spent approximately two years studying and then teaching as an assistant with the Arica Institute, which offered a variety of Buddhist-based practices and unique meditations. And, while my spiritual context broadened, my original experiences remained unidentified. While with Arica, I studied with a group of psychic healers who were associated with Edgar Cayce's organization, the A.R.E. (the Association of Research and Enlightenment) and the Science of Mind Church. My training with this group was extensive, led to more teaching, and carried me closer to understanding what I had experienced. However, this learning period was steeped in esoteric belief structure that *for me* over-complicated what I accepted as natural.

I emerged from those years of training with perspective and an understanding that I must draw from myself what I knew and let go of what was not relevant. I decided to move to Boulder, Colorado. This gave me an opportunity to more fully listen to myself and to start a private practice. A synergy of connections and information helped me clarify my original experiences and what context they belonged in.

I knew that our bodies have the ability to experience energy, which I had always called *light*. I also understood that our bodies hold the keys to our consciousness and spiritual awakening. These realizations became the foundation of the healing work I developed. By 1984 my private practice had grown to include teaching and forming a healing school, called the Transformational

Healing Institute. THI served the community by creating a forum for the study of energy healing. Its curriculum included long-term courses in meditation, energetic and psychic self-healing, and karma work. THI also offered practitioner certification programs. These trainings centered on developing proficiency in specific healing techniques, such as the Psychic Cord Release Process^{SM} and the Past Life Resolution Process^{SM}, as well as a number of other transformational practices. I directed the Institute and taught its courses until 1991. It was a powerful time of teaching and learning in which I saw many years of searching and training bear fruit.

Following the seven years that I spent directing THI, I have concentrated on private practice and energy education through individual and group mentoring.

Where Body Meets Soul

Every student and client I have ever worked with has prepared me to write this book. Each one of them has taught me the multiplicity of ways that subtle energy and the energy system mirror our wholeness and the interrelationship between our thoughts, emotions, actions, health, and innate spiritual connectedness. *Where Body Meets Soul* offers the energy education not yet established in our culture and provides clear guidelines for integrating this learning into daily life through self-care.

Energetic self-care is a process of reinstating and/or maintaining wholeness – a reaching inward to a deeper experience of body connection, emotional awareness, sensory awakening, and soul recognition. Unwittingly, most of us have been trained to compartmentalize ourselves. Through broad collective and individual beliefs, we have learned to separate our bodies from our thoughts and emotions and our bodies from our spirits. We have conditioned ourselves and been conditioned to limit our perceptions. We have lost coherence.

As you focus within your energy system and work with your subtle energy, you are literally "connecting the dots" of your body, mind, and soul – bringing physical-spiritual integration to the forefront of your consciousness. This depth of self-connection can be learned *or* reawakened. To do so, you simply need clear information and balanced stages of experiential learning. Therefore, I have designed this book in a course format, which incorporates energetic exercises, *practices*. The practices provide you with an active learning process, which guides you in how to strengthen your energy system – how to nourish it, utilize it, and renew it. However, you do not need to wait for completion of the exercise series to reap benefits. Each practice constitutes an immediate act of self-care – of energy revitalization, clearer connection with self, and increased spiritual and physical well-being.

How to Use This Book

Where Body Meets Soul presents a self-guided instructional program, which can be used by an individual, by partners or friends, or by a group. The book consists of three main sections. The first is the Context, which explores and details the subjects of the energy system, the basics of energetic self-care, and the relationship between energy and transformation. The Context serves as a reference for your experiences with the energetic practices, and it can also stand alone as a clear guide to understanding the seamless interconnection between physicality and spirit.

The second section is the Energetic Practices. These exercises uniquely function as both a series and as individual self-care and self-healing tools. Nine practices, initially used in sequence, form the series. Each exercise includes a suggested time frame for practice, usually one to two weeks. The series sequence, as well as the timetable, supports your energy system to awaken and strengthen at an optimal rate.

The third section, the Integration, provides an in-depth review of the specific benefits, practical applications, challenges, and energetic influences of each practice. Attending to the Integration work that accompanies each exercise will help you develop a broader, working knowledge of subtle energy healing practices and will guide you in more skillfully addressing your ongoing needs for personal growth, transformation, and self-care.

Fulfilling the practice sequence requires some time. The time needed will vary from 10-20 minutes every two or three days. You can determine the number of times per week. However, a minimum of once a week is essential. The entire series will take approximately 15-20 weeks to complete. You may wish to extend the time, but I would not recommend shortening it. **If you would like a shorter program,** I suggest that you work with the first four practices only. Proceeding with the time frame these practices provide, you would complete in six to seven weeks. You may then continue to use them as individual self-care exercises and finish the remaining practices when it is convenient for you.

I strongly recommend that you keep a practice journal to aid you in remembering the details of your experiences. Even minimal journaling can maintain continuity week to week and help you monitor your progress.

To further understand the course work of this book or determine if it suits you at this time, I suggest that you read Care and Strengthening of the Energy System and Energy Gain and Transformation in the Context section.

If you are prone to emotional or psychological disorders or are under professional supervision for such conditions, you should check with your doctor or practitioner to secure outside support. Together you can determine if this work is appropriate for you. **Although these practices are self-care techniques, they are not designed to replace professional medical or psychological care.**

If you are pregnant, do not begin these practices. Your pregnancy is a physical-spiritual process unto itself. The addition of new energetic influences would distract from all that is happening within you and would initiate other changes. If you wish, however, you may choose to read through this material to find important reminders for improving self-care. The introductions to each of the practices and/or the Integration material can encourage you to make corrective behavioral and attitudinal adjustments.

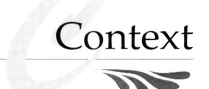

Part I

Context

BODY AND SOUL ARE NOT SEPARATE. THEY RESIDE TOGETHER BRIDGING THE SEEN AND THE UNSEEN WORLDS.

WORKING WITH SUBTLE ENERGY AND THE ENERGY SYSTEM is not yet a common practice in Western, mainstream culture. Consequently, we have no foundational paradigm or shared language to reference these subjects. Nor can most of us turn to our upbringing – family history, public education, and religious training – to source them. We have no context.

The material in this section provides that touchstone. It presents detailed information about the energy system and an overview of the transformational influences of subtle energy on the body and consciousness. The Context is concise and clear, yet, at first read, may present more information than you feel that you need or can easily absorb. Read it once or as often as you desire. Referencing this material while you work with the energetic practices will help you confirm and clarify your experience – and it will help you take greater ownership of what you are learning.

The Unified Field

A common life force energy links us to one another, to the Earth, to the universe. It resonates within us, and it surrounds us – weaving us into the whole of creation, while never diminishing our individual natures. The unified field is the totality of this energy. And all life forms, animate and inanimate, are part of its whole.

The all-encompassing nature of the unified field exposes the sacred paradox of our existence – as physical-spiritual beings we are both individuated and living in a flawless state of Oneness. Each of us navigates this profundity, this dilemma, in our own ways, according to our spiritual and philosophical sensibilities and knowledge.

Subtle energy practices are powerful tools that help us in this endeavor. Through their specific and focused steps, they lead us to resolve the illusionary schisms between body and soul, matter and spirit, and the sacred and the mundane. Subtle energy practices aid us in activating the blueprint of our wholeness, the actual mechanisms that awaken our experience of all that we are – and all that is.

The Human Energy System

The body is physical and it is nonphysical – it is of energy and consciousness. In the same way our physiological systems maintain and regulate the body's varying physical functions, the energy system maintains our energetic functions and sustains our integrated consciousness. It receives, transmits, circulates, and retains life force energy and interconnects the physical, mental, emotional, and spiritual aspects of our living beings. The human energy system consists of the energy field or aura, energy centers called chakras, energy pathways known as meridians, and a central vertical axis or physical channel.

The Aura

The aura is an emanation of subtle energy, which radiates through and from the body and consciousness. The aura emits and carries the energetic frequencies of our thoughts, beliefs, emotions, spiritual qualities, and physical condition. The aura also embodies lingering energy from past lives and the frequencies of our manifesting futures.

The energy of the aura generally extends two to four feet around the body and forms an energy field – an energetic environment and boundary in which we are contained. This container serves to both define and protect us. It distinguishes us and separates us from other energies, keeping us psychically and energetically within ourselves. It is through this containment that we are able to form and maintain self-identity.

Although the aura defines and contains us, it is not static, impermeable, or isolating. The aura expands and contracts; it also connects with and receives other energies. The aura expands in response to our feelings of openness, joy, love, and spiritual experience. It contracts when we are afraid, weak, ill, or negating our personal truths.

The aura naturally connects with and receives energy from the Earth, the unified field, and the energy fields of other people. The aura's link to Earth energy is primarily involuntary, yet can be enhanced or limited by our conscious or unconscious intentions. The aura's connection with the unified field remains constant. However, as individuated beings, our distinct boundaries and filters temper our recognition of it.

When mutual affection and affinity exist between two people, their auras will often join one another – either connecting boundary-to-boundary or fully meshing. The meeting of auric fields is rarely problematic. Their touching feels energizing and subtly stimulating. Once two individuals part, these sensory feelings soon disappear.

When auras mesh, their energy intermingles. When the auras separate, auric energies generally return to their original state. However, in some cases, one or both people may not fully reclaim their energy. As a result, their respective energies become incorporated into the other's aura. The impact of absorbing another person's energy varies. If it is a one-time occurrence, the received energy may "shake off" rather quickly. However, if two people chronically blend energies without reinstating healthy boundaries, they will become enmeshed. Enmeshment can be defined in psychological terms, but it is ultimately an energetic condition.

Our auric energy, whether emitted by us or received, influences both our consciousness and our health. The aura that surrounds us, in part, re-enters us via the chakras and the meridians. It also influences us through its sensory interface with the body, brain, and nervous system. If the aura is weak or filled with confused or life-negating messages and thoughts, it will limit the body and consciousness. If the aura is vital and filled with life-supportive thoughts, emotions, etc., it will be an energetic asset to the body and consciousness.

The auric boundary or border also influences us, protecting our health and well-being by ensuring that our personal energies are contained. When the aura's border is clear and strong, our energies are held intact. When the auric boundary is weak or broken, energy containment is compromised. Energy can leak out or become diffuse. Unwanted energy from others can inadvertently enter. In these cases we are, to varying degrees, weakened physically and muddled emotionally, mentally, and/or spiritually.

The aura and its distinct, yet malleable, boundary are powerful influences in our daily, physical lives. When considered in the context of selfhood and physical-spiritual wholeness, the aura is a perfect mirror. It projects and reflects the energies of who we are. Maintaining a healthy aura is key to our well-being, integrity, identity, and health.

The Chakras

The chakras are energy centers that interconnect the physical body with the aura. The major chakras are located at the perineum, in the pelvis, torso, neck, head, and at the top of the head. The ones in the trunk of the body, neck, and forehead have a front and a back, while all have center points. The chakras are funnel-shaped and extend from within the aura (at their wide end) to the center of the body (at their narrow end). Minor chakras are situated symmetrically on both the right and left sides of the body. The number of identified chakras varies depending on which spiritual or healing modality one uses. Typically in Western practices, seven to nine major chakras are acknowledged. Our course work uses an eight-chakra system.

The chakras receive, transmit, conduct, and retain energy. Through clockwise and counterclockwise spiraling motion, they mediate energy between the auric field, the unified field, other people, and the body. Chakras draw vital energy into the body and nourish its physiological systems. Each chakra has the greatest energetic influence in the area of the body in which it is located and directly affects the health of the nearby organs, musculature, bones, and physiological functions.

Chakras are also consciousness centers. In this capacity, they function as specialized minds, each one overseeing a particular set of life activities and issues. (These are described in detail in the Energetic Practices section.) The chakras open or close, receive, block, and transmit energy according to our internal, often unconscious, responses to experience. They also record and hold the energy of our emotions, beliefs, and history associated with specific events, situations, or relationships. When we are clear and resolved with a particular experience, the corresponding chakra reflects this. The chakra carries, in energy, any wisdom and benefit gleaned from the experience. Chakra health remains stable or improves. However, when a life experience is not resolved and complete, the chakra embodies the incompletion. It retains what has not digested: toxic, stuck, or muddled emotions, trauma, conflicts, thought patterns, and/or any related history. In this case, the chakra's health, energy, and functioning become compromised and the body is burdened.

Since chakras extend from within the aura to the center of the body, a part of our chakras' energy resides in our physical beings. Thus, clear, vital chakra energy creates a vital body area. Blocked chakra energy creates a congested or stagnant body area. Grief, fear, or rage held in a chakra creates a body area that carries these emotions. When dealing with problematic physical conditions, the chakra located in the affected area always carries information about the causal level of the stress or disease. By addressing the causal level, healing is accelerated and chakra balance restored.

The chakras are main energy receivers for our bodies. They also carry records of our life experience. The chakras demonstrate how body, energy, and consciousness interconnect in a dynamic way. Thus, the chakra system offers one of the most potent and obvious links between consciousness and the energetic and physiological conditions of the body.

The Meridians

Energy pathways called meridians form specific flow patterns that carry energy through the body to nourish it and sustain the physiological functions of the organ systems. The main meridians govern the organs: lungs and large intestine, the spleen and stomach, the heart and small intestine, the bladder and kidney, the pericardium and triple burner (glandular system), gallbladder and liver. Auxiliary meridians take over when energy or circulation in the main meridians becomes severely compromised.

The meridians lie at varying levels beneath the skin (more superficial in the hands, feet, and head, deeper in the arms and legs, and deepest in the torso) and have entrance and exit points for energy at the skin's surface. The point of exit of one meridian rests next to the point of entry in the following meridian, creating a continuous circulating pathway around the body. Although energy circulates in each meridian at all times, energy in each main meridian intensifies at certain times of day. The cycles of intensification change every two hours and begin with the liver from 1-3 a.m. and end with the gallbladder at 11 p.m.-1 a.m. (A full chart of times is located in the Appendix.) The periods of intensification are helpful to note because repeated discomfort at these times of day may indicate imbalance in the corresponding meridian.

The traditional method of assessing the energetic condition of a meridian consists of reading its corresponding pulse. Pulse points located on the inner wrists will reveal energetic imbalances such as depletions, stagnations, or hyperactivity. The energetic qualities of an organ and its corresponding meridian will change in response to chakra functioning, as well as overall physical and emotional health and well-being. Meridian changes will also occur in response to climatic conditions, as our bodies and energy interact with the atmosphere that surrounds us.

Food also plays a part in organ and meridian health since food has a variety of energetic influences. For example, food can contain calming, exciting, drying, warming, and/or cooling properties that will directly influence the temperament and tempo of internal energies. Chinese herbal medicine embodies this knowledge and uses herbs as well as food to balance energy and restore meridian and organ health.

Emotions can influence, as well as reflect, organ and meridian wellness. All emotions are part of being human. Emotions arise and move through us in a way that is natural to who we are and the circumstances we are experiencing. However, an overload of emotion can burden an organ system, and a stressed organ system does not facilitate the movement of emotional energy. This interrelationship of body energy and emotion aids us in knowing which meridians are out of balance. Anger corresponds to liver and gallbladder, anxiety and worry to stomach and spleen, fear to kidney and bladder, grief to lung and large intestine, and excitableness and depression to heart and small intestine.

The meridians form a circulation system that transports energy, which inflows at their entrance points and the energy absorbed into the body via the chakras and the aura. The meridians' specificity of function and the extent of their energetic influence provide us with a powerful diagnostic and healing tool.

Please note: The exercises presented to you in this book do not directly address the meridians, but will influence them through overall strengthening of the energy system. The art and science of working with the meridian system comprises the core of traditional Chinese medicine. To more fully understand the science and spirituality of this modality, I recommend that you read *The Complete System of Self-Healing: Internal Exercises* by Dr. Stephen T. Chang and/or *The Web That Has No Weaver: Understanding Chinese Medicine* by Ted J. Kaptchuk.

The Physical Channel

The human body exists in natural relationship with the Earth and the sky – with form and formlessness. Within the energy system this relationship is reflected by the first chakra (at the perineum) and the seventh chakra (at the top of the head). The first chakra opens to the Earth and primarily governs issues of physical security and survival. The seventh opens to the sky and governs our connectedness to the Infinite. The central axis that lies between these two poles, in line with the center points of the major chakras, is the physical channel.

The body as a physical form stands in a vertical position on the Earth. As energy flows from the Earth upward and from the sky downward, ascending and descending energies support the body and consciousness. A balance of these energies has a favorable effect on the spine, joints, musculature, nervous system, and chakras. Balance, in regard to these energies, means that descending energy has not overtaken the body and weighed it down, nor has ascending energy overwhelmed the body causing it to be top-heavy and ungrounded. Further, equilibrium between the first and seventh chakras affects one's consciousness as well, balancing one's relationship to form and formlessness, physicality and spirit.

Ascending energy conducted through the physical channel provides a unique source of healing and transformation. When we intentionally focus on this upward movement, the body is lifted internally. The spine elongates and muscles gently stretch and relax. Spiritually, our inner reality is also affected. As energy ascends, it travels from form (first chakra) to formlessness (seventh chakra). As the body lifts, tension patterns created by defensive, fearful, and egocentric attitudes are released – sent into formlessness. We are refreshed and left with an undeniable sense of peace and openness.

An energized physical channel also promotes a greater level of spiritual-emotional-sexual integration. Sex at the energetic level unites the auras, chakras, and physical channels of two people, thus allowing their consciousness and subtle energies to directly interconnect. When the physical channel is open and strong, the flow of all energy improves. Deep emotions within the heart chakra, as well as sexual and spiritual energies, are freer to circulate in the energy system and be exchanged between partners. Sexuality then becomes a cooperative act of pleasure and transformation having great healing potential physically, energetically, and spiritually.

The physical channel is a powerful resource and ally in maintaining our wholeness. Its relationship to the first and seventh chakras promotes the balance of physical and spiritual consciousness. It teaches us how to be in the physical world, without being over-identified with it. It is the stable core of who we are.

Care and Strengthening of the Energy System

When we are children, our parents and caretakers concern themselves with our health. We are taught ways to eat, rest, and exercise. We are taught proper hygiene and daily maintenance of our bodies. Likewise, most of us receive some form of early religious education or practice to help guide and comfort us in this world. From these foundations, we continue to learn how to best sustain our bodies and our lives.

In most of our upbringings, however, energy was never acknowledged. As a result, we do not understand its connection to our bodies, its influence on our health and consciousness, or its role in our spiritual lives. Filling this void in our collective education is easily possible and, in fact, it is essential. With the body's energy system as a guide, we can experience our own energetic natures, learn to utilize our greater consciousness capabilities, and more effectively nurture our physical-spiritual well-being and wholeness.

To begin this education we must first consider the basic needs of the energy system: nourishment, rest, renewal, and exercise.

The required nourishment of the energy system is energy. Energy comes through many sources in our lives: food, emotions, thoughts, activity, relationships, and environment. Energy, in relation to food, refers to the life force and vitality of food itself – not the caloric content and conversion. Energy also comes from nutrient value, as well as the intangible influences of those who grow and prepare the food. Everything we choose to eat and drink either nourishes, fails to nourish, weakens, or damages our energy and our physical bodies.

Emotions and thoughts carry energy. They either nourish, fail to nourish, drain, or damage who we are. Use of life force – work, play, spiritual practice, creativity, etc. – directs energy that nourishes, fails to nourish, drains, or damages who we are.

Relationships – deep, connected relationships, family relationships, sexual relationships, and relationship with self – all generate their own brand of powerful energy that either nourishes, fails to nourish, drains, or damages who we are.

We receive and absorb energy from our environment. We take in energy through breath. We receive energy from nature, people, our surroundings, and the mental-emotional atmosphere in which we live. Our environment nourishes, fails to nourish, drains, or damages who we are.

Rest and renewal of the energy system is imperative to our health and well-being, because depletion of vital energy can lead to physical debilitation and illness. Rest, in this case, does not refer to a ceasing of the activity of the energy system. It means that overuse or misuse of life force energy needs to stop. Only then can one's focus shift to a receptive state of being so that a natural inflow of energy can occur.

Renewal of the energy system refers to the clearing, replenishing, or rebalancing of a chakra(s), the aura, a meridian(s), and/or the physical channel, ideally done on a regular basis, rather than a crisis-directed one.

Exercise of the energy system entails using practices that strengthen its functioning. Subtle energy healing practices as well as tai chi, qi gong, yoga, and many forms of martial arts awaken the energy system and increase its energetic capacity.

Throughout the practice series in Part II, you will learn to nourish, rest, renew, and exercise your energy system. In doing so, you will gain energy and increase your capacity to receive, transmit, conduct, and retain energy. This expansion will be accomplished through step-by-step development, much like physical conditioning would require. Energy gain, made in appropriate increments, allows your energy system to strengthen at a comfortable, natural pace.

Energy Gain and Transformation

For most of us, direct energy gain is a new experience and may initially bring a number of interesting results. Ironically, at times energy gain can create a feeling of fatigue. This response occurs in those of us who run on adrenaline, caffeine, nicotine, or sugar, and/or are lacking proper rest. The energy received from energetic practices exposes the actual energy baseline of the body, and we finally feel our exhaustion. Learning how to rest, receive energy, and better nourish the energy system are the best ways to rebalance and neutralize this reaction.

In response to energy gain, we may at times feel giddy and somewhat euphoric. This response is temporary and of no lasting consequence. The euphoria tends to follow practices that access the subtle energy of the seventh chakra. A lack of grounding can result if a person does not completely absorb the energy gain after the exercise. There are simple directions included in this book that will quickly re-balance this condition.

Sometimes energy gain motivates us to dance all night, work harder, or in some way use up the energy we have gained. This response occurs in those of us who are not used to absorbing and retaining energy. We feel that when we have energy, we must use it. This tendency can also be easily corrected. You will find guidelines for doing so in the Energetic Practices.

When we absorb and retain energy gain, we can often relieve ourselves of weakening chronic conditions such as backache, fatigue, and allergies. Food cravings and a variety of addictions may also end as a result of energy absorption. I have seen people spontaneously give up chocolate, coffee, cigarettes, and marijuana. These changes can occur at various stages of energetic strengthening.

Psychological, emotional, and spiritual changes occur just as often. Experiences such as a clearer sense of self, better psychological boundaries, identification with one's intrinsic values, and a greater expression of one's will and personal power all typically accompany energy gain. For some of us these changes happen automatically. For others, the changes happen as the result of the intentional healing of self-limiting perceptions, beliefs, and emotional patterns. Through energy gain, we often find the motivation to clean our "psychic-emotional houses" and relieve ourselves of behaviors and attitudes that no longer represent or serve who we are. Energy retained from a particular exercise or through accumulated practice can provide a missing component of our wholeness. Like water that seeks its own level, energy will infiltrate and fill the parts of a person that are experiencing a lack or a void.

Occasionally, movement toward transformation occurs very deep within the body and consciousness in areas that have been hidden or closed for some time. Emotions and feelings connected with unresolved difficult experiences rise to the surface. It is important to give these past experiences a voice and a new prospect for growth and transformation. However, if the past experiences are extremely painful, we may not be able to work with them by ourselves.

If during the course work of this book you feel a need to address deeply held emotions and experiences, be honest about your ability to support yourself. When you need help, do not hesitate to contact a health practitioner or healer adequately qualified to help you in your process. (In the Appendix you will find a resource list that can aid you in finding an appropriate, skilled practitioner.)

The transformation you experience as a result of developing your energy system is always integral to who you are; however, it is often accelerated. Energy is alive; it is the prime mover within and around you. When you cultivate a relationship with energy, you naturally catalyze the parts of yourself that are stagnant. Transformation will result. (The Integration section of this book supports you in the transformational influences of the practices.)

The Energy System and Meditation

Energy is mutable and so is your energy system. When any part of you alters in quality or condition, your energy system immediately reflects it. The complement is also true. When any part of your energy system awakens, strengthens, or weakens, your body, mind, and soul are affected. When you understand this and work with the energy system in an informed way, you are able to intentionally and specifically influence change within yourself.

Many ancient healing and spiritual traditions embodied this knowledge and utilized practices that focused on the energetic aspects of the body. Through energy practices, shamans and spiritual practitioners experienced transcendent states of consciousness, maintained their health, healed others, fulfilled their spiritual goals, and enjoyed extraordinary connectedness between the physical and nonphysical worlds. Today, such practices are still upheld in certain domains of tradition. They are also available in secular culture in apportioned forms through practices such as yoga, Chinese energy medicine, and certain meditation techniques.

Meditation is a broad term, encompassing a variety of practices ranging from energetic healing techniques to creative visualizations. Each form of meditation has specific techniques and goals, while incorporating the intention of experiencing a clearer state of awareness or heightening of consciousness. However, beyond the characteristics that define meditation practices and styles, it is important to remember that meditation is a natural energetic and physiological experience.

Spontaneous states of meditation can occur when you are deeply focused. You might be enjoying the beauty and serenity of nature, listening to a sublime musical performance, or feeling strongly connected to someone or something you love. Your body relaxes. Your brainwave patterns change, as do your pulse and respiratory rates. Pleasurable feelings, such as openness, receptivity, peace, or completeness, follow. Elevated sensory experience and transcendence are also common. (Transcendence refers to awareness beyond the range of normal waking consciousness and ego identity.)

The energetic practices in this book offer you step-by-step instruction in how to awaken, nourish, and strengthen your energy system. Through their use you will re-establish coherence between your body, mind, and soul, enjoy deeper levels of relaxation, and more readily experience transcendent states of awareness. And, therefore, at times during the practice series, you will meditate.

Your meditation will vary from light to deep levels and will begin at the moment that your body and mind listen as one to your energy system. Your ability to listen will come when it is perfectly right for you and will occur spontaneously, seamlessly connected to your energetic experience.

Part II

Energetic Practices

COMMITMENT TO SELF IS THE FOUNDATION.

WE ARE PHYSICAL-SPIRITUAL BEINGS, yet most of us live outside the conscious experience of this unity. Collectively as well as individually, we seem to have lost entry into ourselves – into a fully inhabited experience of wholeness. The energetic practices in this section invite you to re-enter yourself – to reach beneath the varied, perhaps hurried, activities of your life and meet yourself *as you truly are* physically, emotionally, mentally, spiritually, and energetically. This intimate and restorative contact will awaken you, and your energy system will guide you to better care for yourself.

Thoroughly reading the following introductory material will help you glean the most from this learning and reconnecting process.

Course Format

Initially the exercises are to be practiced one at a time and in sequence. This format allows you to progress step-by-step using each practice as a building block for a specific aspect of energetic awareness and self-care. A suggested practice timetable ensures that you have an adequate number of days to integrate your experience. You use the Integration section in conjunction with the exercises to help you further understand your energy system, to learn to apply the exercises for self-healing, and to recognize new ideas, insights, and/or behaviors that result from your practice.

If you find that you need or want more time than the schedule advises, allow yourself to extend the practice period. However, I do not recommend that you extend it longer than an additional two weeks, as you may lose the rhythm of the developmental process.

As stated in the Introduction, the entire series will take 15 to 20 weeks to complete. If you prefer a shorter sequence at this time, simply practice the first four exercises only. They offer you a reduced, yet complete program of energetic self-care. If you choose this option, I recommend that you still keep to the timetable provided for Practices I – IV.

As you proceed through the practice series, you may find that you simply do not respond to a specific exercise. In this case, I suggest that you continue to practice it, although you may wish to do so less frequently. Keep to the shortest suggested timetable and read the corresponding Integration section as directed, but do not concern yourself with the results. Eventually, a leap in experience and practice will occur that will carry you far beyond any current dislike or challenge with an exercise.

Keeping a Journal

Following each exercise, you will find a set of questions to answer. It is important to use them at least the first two times you practice an exercise. The questions provide a checklist, a means by which you can identify your level of ease or challenge with each practice. Answering the questions will also help you recognize your energetic experiences and track your own developmental process. A journal or notebook is a perfect place to record your responses.

Keeping a journal establishes a grounded way for you to maintain intimate contact with yourself. It gives you an avenue for inner dialogue – a place to think on paper and explore the transformational outcome of the practices. The moments you spend writing will help you turn your attention inward.

Please note: If you practice the exercises with a friend or a group, I recommend that each of you first answer the questions in your journal. After your personal writing is complete, you can then share with each other. Following this suggestion will help you remember more of your immediate experience with the practices.

Your Sitting Posture

In order to open the energy system and enhance the flow of energy in your body, most of the energetic practices require that you sit in an upright position. To gain the most benefit from this seated position, your pelvis needs to be kept higher than your knees. This slight elevation allows the pelvis to tip and your first chakra to open, which creates a strong physical and energetic foundation and helps the spine align properly. This posture can be accomplished when sitting on the floor, on a stool, or in a chair.

If you choose to sit on the floor, you will need a thick cushion, two pillows, or a pillow that can be folded to create suitable height. Sit on the edge of your cushion, rather than sitting full on. Hanging off the cushion in this way allows the pelvis to tip. You may then cross your legs trying to keep your knees on the ground. You can accomplish this by sitting in a lotus position or a half-lotus position. The lotus and half-lotus are yoga postures that bring the feet (or one foot) over the top of your legs (leg).

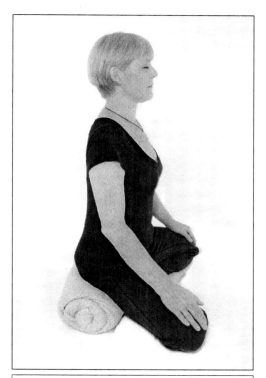

Another position that works well is tucking one foot into your groin area and placing the other, with the sole turned upward, along your opposite shin. Using this form will automatically widen your sitting position and create a strong triangular foundation. You may also sit on a pillow wedged behind your knees. In this case your shins are resting on the floor. You can, likewise, use a Japanese-style meditation bench.

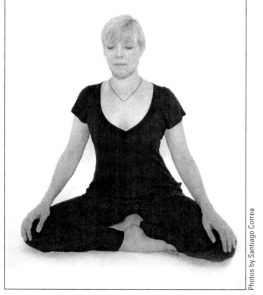

Photos by Santiago Correa

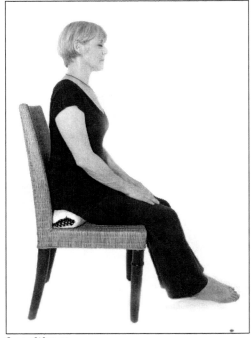

Sitting in a chair is an equally good option. This especially helps if you have stiff leg muscles or hip, back, or knee problems. A wooden or an erect upholstered chair will work well. In either case, placing a folded pillow just under your hips, *not* under the back of your thighs, will help you achieve the desired posture and keep your knees lower than your pelvis.

No matter what sitting method you decide to use, you will find that over time your body will become stronger and more comfortable during sitting. In the meantime, do not hesitate to move your leg positions or support your back during an exercise in order to keep yourself free from discomfort.

Please note: If you have any physical condition or disability that restricts you from sitting, proceed with the exercises in a position that is comfortable and that still allows you to remain alert.

Where to Practice

Where you practice your energy exercises needs to be pleasant, uncluttered, relatively quiet, and calm. I recommend that you practice in a place in your home where you will not be interrupted by other people or by the phone. I also recommend that you choose a place you enjoy – your bedroom, a favorite spot in your living room, or a place near a garden window. If you are fortunate enough to have an extra room in your home, you may want to consider setting up a dedicated practice space. This room can serve as a physical sanctuary – a space that you design and decorate to enhance your energetic experiences.

Although the place you choose in your home will influence your practice, your practice will also influence the place. As you work with the exercises, you will begin to emanate clearer and stronger energy. This revitalized energy will change the feel and energetic quality of the area and room in which you are seated. Therefore, you will find that over time the place where you consistently practice will become an energetic asset to you. Your body and energy system will respond more quickly there. You may also find that merely sitting in this place begins to awaken you energetically.

Please note: Until you have completed the entire self-care series, do not practice any exercise outdoors – except for the one that clearly directs you to do so. Being indoors will help you to learn to focus internally. Upon completing the practice series, your connection with your own energy system will be strong enough for you to successfully practice these exercises anywhere, whether it is quiet or not.

Trust, Focus, and Intention

Your body and energy system are energetic instruments. They are designed to do the very thing that each exercise requires. Interlinked to them, your unconscious awareness recognizes energy on a constant basis. As you enter this energetic practice series, trust the faculties of your body, energy system, and unconscious awareness. They are your allies; they will understand and fulfill the directions you give them.

The energetic practices require that you consciously connect with yourself. This contact happens through your ability to focus. To initiate self-connection, each exercise will direct you to focus in a particular way. Usually you will be asked to place your attention in the physical center of your heart chakra. At other times you may need to focus on the soles of your feet or perhaps your first chakra.

Focus is not a form of visualization, but rather an intentional connection made with the body and/or energy system *that is palpable.* When you focus within yourself, you will most likely notice a sensation – physical or energetic. This sensation confirms *contact.* If you do not feel a specific sensation when you focus, you may notice a sudden release of tension or begin breathing more deeply. These too are signals of connection. Over time and with practice, more direct sensations will come.

Although focusing may challenge you initially, continue to practice. Each intentional connection you make will strengthen your awareness of your body and energy system. As you proceed through the practice series, you will find that focusing in the body and energy system provides a clear, grounded, and refreshing way to enter energetic practice and, eventually, meditation.

After making contact within yourself through focusing, you will need to communicate directly with your body, energy system, and levels of your unconscious awareness. Primarily, this is accomplished through an affirmative intention or verbalization.

Your energy and your energy system are aware, intelligent parts of you. They are activated by and respond to your conscious and unconscious thoughts, emotions, intentions, and declared directions. The practices presented in this section rely on this natural form of internal communication. In different ways throughout the series, you will be asked to state or hold an intention. As you do so, your energy and your energy system will respond accordingly. You do not have to force the direction, nor do you need to doubt it. Your body, mind, and energy system will follow the course that you set. This is how *it always works*.

Practices I – III

The first three practices in the series focus on your daily and habitual uses of energy. They address issues of receptivity, conservation of energy, energetic boundaries, and the interconnectedness of body and consciousness. These self-care exercises are simple yet powerful, challenging the self-limiting beliefs and behaviors that drive you to drain or misuse your energy. Practices I – III will help you *re-gather* yourself and establish an internal equilibrium that is the foundation of subtle energy health. At this beginning facet of practice, open your heart to yourself.

I.
Self-Nurturing Meditation

The energy system serves your body, mind, and soul by receiving, conducting, transmitting, and conserving life force energy. Receptivity, in this context, is vital to maintaining physical health as well as emotional and spiritual well-being. Receptivity can be understood as the ability to *take in* – take in life experience, support, love, energy, and self. To be receptive is to be self-nurturing.

Meditation

Close your eyes and take two or three gentle cleansing breaths, inhaling very slowly through your nose and exhaling very gently and slowly out of your mouth.

Now, focus your attention in the physical center of your heart chakra. *This chakra is located approximately one to two finger-widths above the base of your sternum. Focus inward from this point and as close to the core of your body as is comfortable for you.*

In your own words, speaking internally to yourself:

Affirm your intention and commitment to love and support yourself.

Affirm your responsibility as a creative force in your own life.

Forgive yourself for any pain and difficulty you have created for yourself.

Now, just as you would love and support a dear friend who needed healing, be willing to love yourself in the same way.

Hold yourself in your heart chakra and call the love and compassion that you would give outwardly back into your own heart chakra.

Continue to hold yourself and receive your love. *Hold this receiving focus for as long as you wish.*

When you are ready, ask yourself *what you need* and listen in your heart for the answer. When you hear your response, make a commitment to meet this need.

Gently release your focus when you are ready and open your eyes.

Questions to answer in your journal:

1. What did you feel emotionally during the meditation?

Handwritten margin notes:

- Breathe
- Heart Chakra
- Affirm
- Forgive
- Hold yourself
- Call love to heart ♡

- Hold,
- Receive

Then ask...
- What do I need?
- Listen in heart to answer

2. Did you have any trouble affirming the statements in your heart?

3. Did you feel love and/or energy flow back into you? Did you experience receiving?

4. What was your need? Do you have any resistance to meeting that need?

5. Write down any other feelings and experiences you had during the meditation.

Practice Support: After practicing this meditation and answering the questions listed above, I recommend that you practice the meditation one or two more times *during the practice period* before turning to the corresponding material in the Integration section. Each time you practice, I would suggest that you briefly journal about the experience. You may again use the questions as a guide.

If you find that you do not feel love or energy flowing into you, continue on to the following supplemental exercise, Hands Over Heart. Feel free to practice it in conjunction with this meditation, or in place of it, as needed.

Difficulty with receiving energy or love back into the heart can come from chronic stress or immediate life circumstances. It may also be part of a long-standing energetic and emotional habit pattern. Whatever the cause of the difficulty, be assured that you will be able, given enough time, to heal the situation. Reading the Integration material may help you uncover and deal with the cause.

Integration for this practice begins on page 93.

Recommended practice time for the Self-Nurturing Meditation is 2 weeks. Practice this exercise at least 5 times within the two-week period. You may then wish to use an abbreviated version in which you simply hold yourself in your heart.

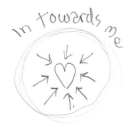

In towards me

Hands Over Heart

This exercise is simple and direct. It can be used when you are having difficulty receiving energy into your heart in the Self-Nurturing Meditation or any time you are under a great deal of stress. It does not require effort or focus on your part. Placing your hands over your heart center (chakra) is soothing and calming. It supports you while gently flowing energy into your body.

Exercise

Close your eyes and focus your attention physically in your heart chakra.

Place your hand(s) over this chakra and be attentive to the feeling of energy flowing inward into your heart center.

Hold this focus for as long as you like.

Release the focus and open your eyes when you are ready.

Questions to answer in your journal:

1. Does having your hands over your heart feel supportive and comfortable?
2. Were you able to feel energy flow into your heart?
3. Did your body sigh and inhale?
4. Do you feel more relaxed?

Practice Support: The desired result of this exercise is that you are able to feel energy flowing gently inward into your heart. If this happened, you can discontinue this exercise for now and proceed with the Self-Nurturing Meditation.

If this exercise has not produced the desired result, I encourage you to continue with it, giving yourself an extended opportunity to awaken the receiving capacity of the heart. You can read the

Integration section that corresponds with the Hands Over Heart exercise at any time.

Integration for Hands over Heart begins on page 97.

II.
Inflow Exercise

In the course of your daily activity and work you likely exert a great deal of energy. You focus on the job at hand. You complete your to-do lists and fulfill your external commitments to your children, your spouse, extended family, career, and community. Energetically speaking, you are exhaling. *You are in outflow.* An emphasis on expending energy, rather than receiving and conserving it, depletes you physically, mentally, emotionally, and spiritually. The antidote for energy depletion is retrieval and inflow.

Exercise

Close your eyes and focus attention in your body.

Take time to notice and be aware of the energy that you give out. Give yourself time to review your day, your week. Notice what in your life has recently required a great deal of your energy.

Now, in your heart, ask your outflowing energy to gently flow back into you. *If the energy flow seems uncomfortable or too strong, place your hands over your heart and that will help regulate the flow of energy.*

From time to time, notice how your body feels. If your body is tense, soften your stomach area and take one or two slow, deep breaths. This will support your body in receiving the inflowing energy.

Continue this process until you feel complete. (3-10 minutes)

Gently release your focus and intention. Open your eyes.

Questions to answer in your journal:

1. How do you feel physically, energetically, and emotionally?
2. Were you able to feel the inflow of your energy? If so, did it feel good, comfortable? If you were not comfortable, did placing your hands over your heart help you?
3. If you were unable to inflow your energy, were you consciously aware of any concerns about doing so?
4. Write about all other feelings or experiences that you had during this practice.

Energy gain and body feedback:

After completing this exercise, wait approximately 20 minutes and notice how you are feeling. If you feel a little "top-heavy" or headachy, it means that you are not absorbing all of the energy you have gained. If this is the case, please close your eyes and ask that <u>excess energy</u> release out your tailbone into the Earth. It is important that you say and intend that <u>only</u> excess energy release; then all the energy that you can easily utilize will remain.

Practice Support: Your intention with this practice is to inflow your energy. If you have difficulty with this, relaxing your stomach and placing your hands over your heart chakra are the most helpful adjustments you can make. If after completing three more practices, you continue to be unable to inflow energy, you may replace this exercise with either of the two preceding exercises.

Read the Integration material as soon as you are interested in doing so. It will give you other practical applications for this exercise that you can also practice during the recommended time period.

Integration for this practice begins on page 99.

The recommended practice schedule for this exercise is 1-2 weeks. Practice it at least 3 times during this practice period.

III.
Clearing and Sealing the Auric Field

Before beginning this exercise, review the material about the aura found in the Context section of the book.

The aura is multidimensional in nature and function. It is the energetic container for both the body and the consciousness. It is also one of the key energetic supports for the nervous system and is essential to the maintenance of individual identity. One of the requirements for maintaining a healthy auric field is having a clear, intact boundary.

A strong aura boundary is smooth and defined. A compromised one will look diffuse, frayed, or cracked at the edges. A weak auric boundary may be a temporary or basically benign condition originating from an acute illness or an unusual, energetic response to stress. A chronically frail or a broken boundary, however, may be the result of emotional trauma, debilitating illness, a surgery, or drug or alcohol abuse. Whether the boundary weakness is a temporary or severe condition, the aura will benefit from corrective energy work.

Although improving some conditions in the auric field can be complex, strengthening the quality of the auric boundary is straightforward. Clearing and Sealing the Auric Field is a method of preventing and gently correcting a compromised aura.

Exercise

Before proceeding with this exercise close your eyes and take a few moments to sense your auric field. *This is truly as simple as sensing the space around your body.*

When you are ready to continue, begin by taking two or three deep breaths – breathing in slowly through your nose and exhaling slowly and gently out your mouth.

47

Now, focus your attention in your heart chakra.

Take a few moments to feel your auric field again. This time notice who and what you are carrying too close to you – identify specific people, situations, and concerns.

In your heart, affirm your willingness to release from your aura whomever and whatever is not really a part of you.

From deep within your center, release these people, situations, and concerns. Allow them to leave your immediate space. If necessary, *escort them* all the way out of your auric field.

When you feel complete with this part of the process, place a membrane-like seal around your aura. *Make sure that you have allowed enough space for yourself and have not brought the seal too close to your body. Trust your sense of what feels good to you.*

If you are using this exercise after having a recent surgery, proceed as follows: Initially place the seal quite a distance from your body – about 5 feet away. As you continue to practice this exercise over the practice period, bring the auric boundary in a little closer every 3-5 days until you reach what feels like the best "normal" size. *These steps are necessary, because during surgery your auric field was torn and, due to anesthesia, it has likely also expanded. Sealing the auric field after surgery is very important. However, doing it in small steps is always advised.*

Proceeding with the exercise – if you wish, fill the space inside the seal with light or your favorite color. *Remember that light and color are energy. Be open to what feels good. If you choose a color that is not particularly supportive, it will likely change spontaneously. Accept what feels the best. If you wish to use light, I would recommend trying pure gold light first as it is universally strengthening and protecting.*

Remain in your sealed aura for as long as you wish.

When you are ready, gently release your focus and open your eyes.

Questions to answer in your journal:

1. How do you feel? What difference do you notice?
2. Did you have any difficulty releasing people, situations, and concerns from your aura?
3. Did you feel your seal? Does it feel supportive?
4. Did you use color or light in your aura? How did that work?
5. Record any other experiences and feelings you had during the exercise.

Practice Support: I recommend that you practice this exercise at least two times before reading the Integration section. However, if you feel reluctant about releasing people or situations out of your aura, reading the integration material now may be helpful.

The energy gain with this exercise is likely to be easily absorbed, so you probably will not have to release any excess energy.

Integration for this practice begins on page 101.

Recommended practice schedule is 2 weeks. Practice a minimum of 5 times within the two-week period. If you find that you no longer need to release anybody or anything, just place a seal around your aura and use color or light within the seal if you wish.

Transition to Practice IV

In the course of your day-to-day life, relationship with self can easily shift into autopilot and become governed by beliefs about who you *should* be, what has worked in the past – perhaps as long ago as childhood – or by your strategies to *fit in*. You might further mask connection to self with compensating addictions and habitual lifestyle patterns.

When you connect with your energy system, you reach beneath autopilot mentality, habits, and addictions – and you connect with *how you really are*. The three meditations you have just completed give you a means to recognize how you are in certain areas. The Self-Nurturing Meditation reveals if your heart is open to self or if your heart is closed. The Inflow Exercise focuses on how you spend your energy and your ability to retrieve it. Clearing and Sealing the Auric Field helps you recognize who and what are compromising your boundaries and energy.

As you have discovered in the Integration section, correcting self-limiting energetic habits brings beneficial changes in consciousness. Every time you take intentional action in the practices – *when you hold yourself in your own heart chakra, when you inflow your energy back to yourself, when you seal your auric field with only you inside of it* – you initiate new, supportive behaviors and attitudes.

Practice IV, Chakra Clearing and Balancing, builds from these foundations by introducing you to a more direct experience of body-mind-energy interconnection. Studying the chakras gives you greater awareness of your body, as well as of your emotions, beliefs, and your life history. As a result, you may initially feel overwhelmed. Take your time with these exercises and understand that it can take many years to become adept at chakra work.

Whether you have studied the chakra system before or this is your first time, accept that what you learn at this time *is right* for now. Every opportunity you have to work with your chakras will give you valuable information and promote your continued energetic development and body-mind-soul integrity.

IV.
Chakra Clearing and Balancing

Please review the chakra material in the Context before proceeding.

Relationship with your body and energy system is relationship with self. Your body and energy reflect exactly how you are and how you are *digesting* your life experiences. Learning to listen to your body and energy to decode their messages is exceedingly important. It allows you to know yourself and accurately represent yourself in your life, in relationships, and in the world. The chakras are the *minds* of the body and soul. They carry the most definitive and honest knowledge of who you are. Accessing their information is key to maintaining body-mind-soul unity. Savor this time with your chakras and open to deeper levels of yourself.

Chakras and their Governing Issues

Before working with the energetic exercises for the chakras, it is essential to familiarize yourself with the chakra locations, the life issues each governs, and the physical areas of the body they influence. As you read through this material, make note of the issues that have been most relevant in your life. At the end of this section, you will have an opportunity to review your findings and further identify which chakras most reflect your life focus and challenges.

• **First Chakra,** sometimes called the root chakra, is located at the perineum (between the anus and the genitals). The center point of the first chakra is between the pubic bone and the coccyx. Physical areas most directly influenced are the genital-rectal area, male reproductive system, the bladder, and the coccyx, as well as the legs, knees, and feet.

The first chakra opens to the Earth and primarily governs issues of your physicality and the drives and instincts of your human animal nature.

Physical survival/survival of the ego: Activities and impulses that focus on self-preservation. Confidence in or fear about one's ability to survive and be safe.

Connections with people or things that one equates with self-preservation – one's mate in a security-based relationship; one's business or money.

Instinct or knowing from one's animal nature or cellular level: Urges and impulses that inform us, such as, a sense of danger; sense of direction; ability to recognize truth and lies; psychic and energetic alertness; gut-level recognition.

Sexuality as procreation and/or survival: Physically oriented sexuality or sexual impulse that is not relationship focused. Establishing security, safety, power, position, and/or dominance through sex. *This can be an unconscious drive in any or all sexual experiences and attractions.*

Physical vitality: Being in your body; physical enjoyment; physical presence; strength and capacity; being grounded in the here and now. Feeling connected to the Earth.

• **Second Chakra is located three to four finger-widths below the navel. The center of this chakra is positioned midway between this point and the sacrum. Physical areas most directly influenced are the female reproductive organs, the large intestine and colon, and the sacral area. All bones and musculature in the pelvic area are also affected.**

The second chakra governs connectivity – your openness to merge with others and also with certain energetic experiences. Paradoxically, it also governs your ability to separate and maintain self-connection and boundaries. (Keeping clear boundaries is also a function of the third chakra.)

Energetic and emotional connectedness and merging: Openness to sensation physically and energetically; absorbing or being absorbed by a person or an experience; personal boundary issues; sexual attractions and longing; emotional bonding (along with the heart chakra); sexual union; release to orgasm.

Relationships that have a sexually based or bloodline origin (lovers, parent/child, relatives): Relationships that involve a deep-level and/or cellular connectedness.

Deep feelings of nurturing and sustaining: Visceral urges to nourish and foster the well-being of others; giving one's energy to another; *also, reserving energy for self.*

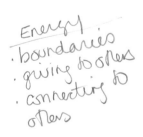

Energy
· boundaries
· giving to others
· connecting to others

Visceral and sexual power and chi center: Self-containment; magnetism; charisma; strong self-identity and boundaries; core strength; self-empowerment; interpersonal power sharing (or power struggles). *Consider that energy is a resource. It can be shared or reserved. When personal energy becomes entangled with others and self-containment is lost, power struggles often result.*

- **Third Chakra is located between the ribs in the diaphragm area (solar plexus) approximately three finger-widths below the base of the sternum. The chakra's center is midway between this point and the spine. Physical areas most directly influenced are the liver, gallbladder, stomach, spleen, small intestine, pancreas, kidneys, and the lumbar vertebrae.**

    The third chakra expresses "I am a self" and governs your drive to affirm and represent self – joyously, honestly, and purposefully.

    Self-acceptance: Self-recognition, self-acknowledgment, and internal validation.

    Conscious connection to one's wants, needs, and emotions: The ability to feel and recognize oneself emotionally; the ability to address one's personal wants, needs, and requirements in life – care of self.

    Self-advocacy: Accurately representing yourself to others and the world at large; supporting personal needs, wants, and values; maintaining a healthy level of self-interest.

    Participation and action: Commitment to self; taking action to support self; engagement – being a part of life.

    Self-esteem that comes from being oneself: Personal fulfillment and enjoyment; confidence; sense of presence (along with the second and first chakras); healthy pride and sense of self-worth.

- **Fourth Chakra is located approximately one to two finger-widths up from the base of the sternum. The center of this chakra rests midway between this point and the spine. The physical areas most directly influenced are the heart, lungs, the upper arms, the breasts, and the mid, as well as low, thoracic vertebrae.**

The fourth chakra, also known as the heart chakra, is the soul center and consequently influences your ability to savor life's greatest joys and resolve its most severe challenges. Love is a core expression of the heart chakra.

Love for oneself and others: The ability to connect with and value the inherent nature of oneself or another.

Compassion and emotional acceptance of oneself and others: The ability to hold a safe space for the temperament and process of self or another; the development of both unconditional love and empathy.

Soul force center or psychic center: The reference point for soul-level discernment; inner gateway to the soul's energy; deep-level seeing and knowing.

Integration and transmutation: The place of ultimate integration of life experience; the soul's cauldron of transmutation and spiritual digestion where all is accepted and turned into knowledge, wisdom, peace, forgiveness, and/or release.

- **Fifth Chakra is located at the fourth cervical vertebrae. The center point is positioned forward from this point in the throat. The physical areas most directly influenced are the neck, throat, larynx, thyroid, jaw, mouth, and cervical vertebrae. The ears can be influenced.**

The fifth chakra is extraordinary in scope, having the ability to allow or dam the flow of energy in other chakras and the body.

Self-expression and communication: Allowing *what is inside the self* to be felt and expressed; giving voice to self; openness to interaction and communication between the physical and nonphysical dimensions.

Creative center: The transcendent experience of creating. Where personal energy and the energy of the Infinite interface to bring ideas, visions, dreams, etc., into manifestation. Creative genius. Creative flow.

Will: The overseer of self and choice. The on-off switch for energy and creativity expressed through allowing or controlling, respecting or negating and judging. *Consider how you feel when you criticize yourself or force yourself to do what is not right for you. Notice your throat. Is it tight, stiff, or blocked? Also, notice your throat when you are being yourself and expressing who you are.*

- **Sixth Chakra is located in the area of the mid-forehead. The center point is inward from the forehead surface approximately two to four inches. The physical areas most directly influenced are the eyes, the sinuses, the brain, and the pituitary gland.**

3rd Eye
· Reflective mind
· See what is... in this and other dimensions

The sixth chakra is the seat of the peaceful, reflective mind. It can be imaged as a still, clear mountain lake whose water mirrors the clouds above it and the peaks that surround it.

Knowing on a spiritual level: Knowing based on a deep, integrated experience of one's true self; inner peace.

Mental clarity: The mind acting in a contemplative, receptive manner; the ability to know *what is.*

Vision: Ability to see in this dimension and beyond; the ability to see *what is.*

- **Seventh Chakra is located at the top of the head. The center point is *above* the body about five to twelve inches above the center of** the head. (The exact location varies from person to person and can be easily discerned. Working with the Chakra Revitalization Exercises and the Heart and Crown Meditation will help you identify this place.) The physical areas most directly influenced are the spine, joints, the brain, the pineal, and the cervical vertebrae.

The seventh chakra, also known as the crown chakra, opens upward to the sky and connects you with the universe, your God, and what is not yet manifested.

Connection with the Infinite: Energetic openness to the nonphysical dimension, transcendent experience, and to what one refers to as *infinite*. Keeping spiritual awareness and values in one's consciousness.

Openness to grace: Experiencing connection to the Infinite as a part of one's day-to-day life process and movement. Feeling spiritually connected and supported.

Release into greater identity: Accepting one's identity as infinite rather than finite. Faith in what lies beyond the ego.

The future: Awareness of what is moving toward manifestation.

• **Eighth or Thymus Chakra is located about one third of the way down from the top of the sternum. The chakra's center is positioned midway between this point and the spine. The physical areas most directly influenced are the heart, lungs, thymus, and the upper thoracic vertebrae. The upper arms and shoulders may also be influenced.**

The thymus chakra governs your ability to relate to and resonate with light.

Connection and receptivity to light: The willingness and ability to accept light; lightheartedness. *Consider your ability to be light and all that that implies physically, emotionally, mentally, and spiritually.*

Illumination: The experience in the body of changing energetic frequency to the extent that the ego-identity or self may transform. Having trust in change and feeling free to fully change. *This chakra assists all levels of your healing.*

Chakras and their governing issues serve as powerful focal points for personal processing and healing. To glean the most from your work with them, take time to consider all the ways any given life experience *speaks to you.* You will see how one life issue or event can activate a number of chakras. For example, personal finances are often connected to concerns of survival and the first chakra. They may be linked to the second chakra – to personal power or interconnection with others. Finances may also be tied to issues of self-esteem and would then be governed by the third chakra. For you, all three chakras could be involved. As you continue to explore the chakra issues, be open to secondary as well as primary influences.

Now take some time to write in your journal. Identify the chakra issues that you find most relevant, emotionally charged, or absent. (An absence of expression within a chakra can indicate an area of great loss or self-denial.) Briefly write about each of the issues you have singled out.

Notice how your body looks and functions. *Do you carry extra weight in a particular area? Is there a part of your body that is chronically stiff or tight? Do you have any damaged vertebrae or areas in your spine that are a source of pain or constant misalignment? Where have your illnesses been centered? Have you had surgeries? If so, where?* Now, link each of your answers to a specific chakra by locating the chakra closest to the affected body area.

Once you have written your responses in your journal, review them and notice which chakras represent or have represented the most challenge in your life. As you proceed now with the energy exercises, make note of how these chakras respond. You may find that they are very energetic and responsive or you may find that they are sluggish or closed. In any case, your energy, body, and consciousness will be informing you – offering you a more complete understanding of your chakra healing needs.

Chakra Revitalization Exercises

Since chakras are energy centers, it is important to know how to connect with them energetically. The two following Chakra Revitalization Exercises offer you specific directions to clear and balance your own chakras. These self-healing exercises can improve chakra health and strengthen your overall energy. They will also aid chronic or acute chakra conditions by initiating consciousness shifts and/or by calming energy imbalances.

When using either of the exercises, **wait three days between practice times.** This three-day period will allow your body and mind to process energetic adjustments occurring in the chakras. Between practices, it is important to listen to your inner process and watch what manifests in your life. You may be able to recognize the consciousness issues that are clearing as a result of your chakra work.

Exercise I – *This exercise works with the center points of the chakras, which ensures that deep issues and chronic energy imbalances will be awakened and made accessible when the time is right for their healing.*

1. Close your eyes and take one or two slow, gentle cleansing breaths. Beginning with the first chakra and working one by one to the eighth, place (through your intention) a white-gold flame in the physical center of

your chakra. As you proceed, verbalize your intention for the flame to clear the chakra. *Notice what you feel. As you become more used to working with this process, you will clearly feel the release. You will likely notice energy leaving the front of your body or a stirring sensation within your body. When the clearing is complete, you will no longer feel such movement. White-gold is a specific light frequency which has potent enlightening, transformational, and transmuting abilities.*

2. After the release feels complete, verbalize your intention that this chakra strengthen and balance. *Balance means that the chakra has an appropriate degree of openness and the ability to respond as needed to life situations and experience.*

3. Once you have completed clearing and balancing all the chakras, take a moment to notice how your body feels. Now, verbally affirm your intention that all your chakras are strong and balanced.

When you complete Exercise I, answer questions 1-4 that follow Exercise II.

Exercise II – *If you were not able to sense the center points of the chakras, or if you have a particularly blocked chakra that needs support, you may prefer this practice. However, if you responded well to the first exercise, continue to use it instead of this one, as working with the center points is preferable.*

1. Close your eyes and take two or three slow, gentle cleansing breaths. Working one by one, beginning with the first chakra and working through to the eighth, consciously intend that energy flow from the back of your chakra through the front of it. As this energy moves, verbalize your intention to clear the chakra. *When you reach the seventh chakra, flow energy through the center above your head.*

2. When the clearing (release) is complete, verbalize your intention that the chakra strengthen and balance.

3. When you have completed clearing and balancing all your chakras, take a moment and notice how your body feels. Now, verbally affirm your intention that all of your chakras are strong and balanced.

Questions to answer in your journal:

1. Did you feel the energy moving in or clearing your chakras?

2. Were you *unable* to feel one or more of your chakras? If so, which ones?

3. Did you feel your chakras strengthen and balance?

4. When you were finished, did you experience a sense of calm and balance?

5. If you practiced both Revitalization Exercises, which method did you prefer?

Practice Support: If you are not experienced at working with the chakra system, I recommend that you take your time with these exercises. As you practice the Revitalization Exercises, you will become clearer about the physical location of each chakra. Making this connection is extremely important, as it will deepen your body-mind-energy relationship.

These exercises will also give you the opportunity to perceive energy by feeling the sensation of it in your body. This will strengthen your understanding of how energy and the physical body interact and how intention influences energy. As you invest time in working with your chakra system, you are laying a new, strong foundation for your own health and well-being.

Wait until after you have completed practicing Exercise I twice or Exercise I and II one time each to read the Integration section.

Integration for all the chakra exercises including phrases begins on page 105.

Recommended time schedule for all the combined chakra exercises including the Chakra Phrases is 2-3 weeks. Please allow 3 days between Revitalization Exercises (even if you are only practicing one of them). It is best to work with your chakras – using Exercise I, II, or the phrases – a minimum of 4 times in the practice period. You can proceed with the Chakra Phrases anytime after you have completed two practices of a Revitalization Exercise.

Chakra Phrases

Healing a chakra most often requires more than energetic work. As consciousness centers, your chakras function as specialized minds – holding and recording your beliefs, uncompleted life experience, and unresolved emotional charges. When you clear a chakra energetically, you release some of its *psychic content*, making the chakra's issues more conscious. If the chakra's content is reasonably current or simple, your chakra can heal and strengthen with energetic work alone. However, when a chakra is compromised by older or substantial unresolved life experience, energy work primarily serves as a catalyst to stir the chakra's records into awareness. In cases of deep chakra imbalances, it is best to continue your healing using emotional, karmic, or psychological processing. You may practice energy exercises, as needed, for additional physical and energetic support.

Although energetic clearing of your chakras often requires process work, conscious examination and resolution of chakra issues alone can completely heal your chakras. The reason for this is very important to understand. Your energy mirrors your consciousness. What you think, feel, or focus on, along with the life experiences you have completed or not completed, governs the energy that resides in you – and specifically in your chakras. When you heal at a consciousness level by releasing self-negating messages, resolving emotional trauma, and/or completing a karmic circumstance, your energy will always clear. And, most amazingly, it happens immediately.

When you practice self-healing, the consciousness aspect of the chakra work can be challenging. The Chakra Phrase Exercise offers a way for you to explore and identify the consciousness issues that relate to a given chakra's imbalance. Through a dialoguing process with your chakras, which involves saying a statement aloud and noticing the energetic response in your chakra, you will be able to recognize specific areas of clarity, confusion, and inner conflict. The following exercise can be used anytime you recognize chronic or acute stress in a chakra area.

Chakra Phrase Exercise

1. Based on your experience with the Revitalization Exercises or how you are currently feeling, choose the chakra you wish to focus on.

2. In your journal or on a piece of paper write the words "open, close, and flutter," horizontally across the top right half of your page, giving each its own column. As you proceed through this exercise, you will be asked to notice if your chakra is responding by opening, closing, or fluttering. You will feel the sensation in your body in the chakra area. **Opening indicates** that the phrase acknowledges your personal truth or agreement with the statement made. **Closing indicates** fear, unwillingness, or conflicting beliefs with the phrase you stated. **Fluttering indicates** confusion, inner conflict, or wavering with the statement.

3. Turn to the page in this book that has the phrases that

correspond with the chakra you have chosen to work with. List the statements vertically down the left half of your paper. (The phrases are on the pages immediately following these instructions). *You may wish to use the statements listed in the book first, then create others that more accurately reflect your life experience. Or, you may prefer to work with your own from the beginning.*

4. First, read the statement silently. Next, close your eyes and say the statement aloud **while focusing on the specific chakra you are working with.** Notice if your chakra opens, closes, or flutters. *Occasionally you will register no response. You may try repeating the phrase. If you still have no response, assume that the statement does not reflect any of your chakra issues.*

5. Open your eyes and check the column that corresponds with your chakra's response: open, close, or flutter.

6. When you have completed all your chakra phrases, review your list to see if you notice any common themes.

7. Answer the questions at the end of the chakra phrase section.

First Chakra

I feel safe and secure.
My instincts are always right.
I feel physically vital and capable.
I will do what it takes to survive.
I am weak.
I am a sexual being.
I know what I know.
I do not feel I can survive_____. (Fill in a specific situation if you wish.)
My instincts will not protect me.

Second Chakra

I have power.

I am willing to nurture myself.

I do not like to connect with people.

_____ has the ability to nurture himself/ herself. (Name a specific person.)

_____ has his/her own power.

I feel connected to _____ , but I do not know how to separate from him/her.

I am a sensual being.

"No."

My power supports and protects me.

Third Chakra

I bring my emotions to the surface.

I do not know what I feel.

I am vulnerable now.

I need _____. (Fill in a need that is currently important to you.)

I let _____ take care of himself/herself.

I act on my own behalf.

I can meet my own needs.

I am angry. (Insert another emotion – afraid, happy, grieving, etc.)

I am angry with_____because_____.

I am ready to take action.

Fourth Chakra

I love and accept myself.

I forgive myself.

I hold my life in my heart.

I love and accept _____. (Name a specific person.)

I forgive _____.

My heart is my home.

My passion for life speaks to me in my heart.

I just don't care anymore.

I hate _____. (Name a specific person.)

I have no peace about _____.

(Fill in a particular situation in your life.)

Fifth Chakra

I need to control myself.

I communicate my feelings freely.

My will is my own.

I let _____ express his/her feelings and
thoughts to me.

I never tell _____ what I truly feel.

I cooperate with others.

I am not creative.

I am in control.

I want to create _____.

I say what I think.

Sixth Chakra

I see *what is*.

I trust my vision.

I need to figure out what is going to happen.

I see my true self.

I feel confused.

My mind accepts what is.

Life is overwhelming.

I feel great peace.

I do not know what is going to happen.

Seventh Chakra (Remember the center of this chakra is above your head – however, you may feel a response or sensation on the top of your head or down your spine.)

> I am one with all life.
> I feel harmony and unity in my life.
> I accept grace and ease in my life.
> I am guided.
> My life is an effort.
> I do not feel I belong.
> I feel ungrounded.
> My body is heavy and difficult to move.
> I feel too open; I feel diffuse.

Eighth or Thymus Chakra

> My body is light.
> I receive light into my heart, into my soul.
> I am unable to change.
> Light connects me with the universe.
> I have no energy.
> My heart is heavy.
> I am able to transform myself.
> I am not worthy of light.
> I can be everything I want to be.
> I am free.

Questions to answer and processing to record in your journal:

1. What phrases caused your chakra to close? to flutter? to open? *You may find that similar phrases have brought the same response. Or, you may discover that what you thought might be a challenge for you is not. The phrases can also reveal an interesting phenomenon – a chakra will open when*

*your truth is spoken even when that truth sounds negative or limiting. For example, a truthful phrase for you and your third chakra could be "I want to take action now," or it could be "I am afraid to take action." In both cases, the truthful phrase will energize and open your chakra. **Personal truth equals energy.** Denial of truth is a form of self-denial and it will always diminish or extinguish energy.*

2. Explore the phrase(s) that caused your chakra(s) to close. Interview yourself about the phrase itself. For example: if your heart chakra closes when you say, "I love and accept myself," you will want to discover *what you do not accept about yourself.* You could also inquire about *why you don't deserve love.* You will likely be able to uncover specific areas of self-judgment and blame. Consider how these issues have played a role in your life currently and in the past. As you wish *or as you need to,* share your discoveries with a friend or discuss them with a qualified therapist. Each "closing" phrase offers potential for considerable growth and inner resolution.

3. Consider the phrases that caused a flutter. Interview yourself as previously suggested. "Fluttering" often reveals places where you are still actively learning or grappling with old beliefs. Listen to yourself and identify, as best you can, the varying pieces of your understanding and/or internal conflict. Explore your history with these issues. You may find that by simply becoming more conscious of these challenges, you make a leap in healing.

4. The phrases that prompted your chakra(s) to open represent your current truth. Consider using them as affirmations to maintain your clarity and focus.

5. Continue to work with additional phrases by creating your own and testing them.

Practice Support: After completing the three stages of chakra work – reading and journaling about chakra issues, practicing the Chakra Revitalization Exercises, and using the phrases – you will have a clearer understanding of the present condition of your chakra system.

At this point in your energetic practice, you do not need to have fully cleared, strong chakras in order to continue with the remainder of the exercises and meditations. You may proceed with confidence if you feel you have opened a dialogue with your body, your chakras, and the issues relevant to you. Your willingness and ability to attend to your chakras on an *ongoing basis* is the goal of this chakra work.

Completion and Transition Point

The completion of Practice IV marks the end of the first phase of energetic exercises. The first four exercises address your personal use of energy and offer you specific ways to establish a more conscious connection with yourself. The overall purpose of these practices is to help you create an energetic foundation to better support your health, well-being, and spiritual potentiality. When you use the exercises in a consistent way, you actively fulfill this purpose.

If you intend to stop the course work at this point, you may begin to use Practices I – IV out of sequence and according to your own needs and preferences. Over a period of time, you will come to know these exercises intimately, and they will become part of you – a part of how you think and how you relate to yourself. Trust yourself and trust your process. In the future, when your time and interest allow, you may continue beginning with Practice V.

If you wish to progress with the practices now, I suggest that you do not use the preceding exercises on a daily schedule. It is best to continue through the series focusing on the current exercise only. This helps you to better recognize the energetic quality of each practice and glean the most from its overall influence.

V.
Heart and Crown
Meditation

The heart chakra governs many levels of your emotional and spiritual awareness. It is the center through which you establish loving and compassionate relationships – with others as well as with self. It is through the heart that you recognize and express unconditional love, the ability to accept and value yourself and others without question or qualifying stipulations.

Unconditional love is a state of heart and mind that is in part transcendent. To reach this level of awareness, you must see beyond the transitory circumstances and façade of the ego and connect with the timeless, spiritual intelligence residing within your soul. The heart chakra, at this depth of consciousness, expresses itself as the soul center, the *spiritual mind* through which you digest life experience and extract its essential meaning.

The seventh chakra, also known as the crown, contains some of the subtlest frequencies within the energy system. The crown governs your openness to the Infinite and energetically carries much of your spiritual awareness and values. It is through your crown chakra that you recognize yourself as an infinite rather than a finite being.

A natural relationship exists between the heart and the crown. The transcendent energy of the deep heart is resonant with the energy and spiritual consciousness of the crown chakra. The refined energy of the crown supports the heart chakra's spiritual purpose. When you intentionally allow the energy of your crown to connect with your heart, your heart chakra energetically lightens and more fully opens to its spiritual depth.

Please note: I recommend that you practice the Heart and Crown Meditation when you have a couple of hours to yourself, *especially the first time you practice it.* The reason for this is that the energy gain from this meditation may be more than you have previously experienced. It is important to have time to integrate this energy properly. After you are more familiar with the energy of the meditation, you will likely not require much time to integrate it.

Preparatory Exercise

Success with the Heart and Crown Meditation depends on your ability to focus your attention in your body in a grounded way. This warm-up exercise gives you a way to practice doing this. **It is important that you practice this warm-up and respect its parameters**, even though it may seem unrelated to meditation and your energy system. If you are not able to keep your focus during this exercise, do not proceed with the Heart and Crown Meditation. Instead, repeat the warm-up daily, until you have developed your ability to focus. As soon as you successfully complete this preparatory exercise one time, **you need never practice it again.**

Exercise

Close your eyes. Focus your attention in your right big toe. Hold your focus right there. Allow yourself to develop a singular concentration *on your toe.*

Now, when you are ready, slowly move your focus of attention from your big toe upward along the side of your foot. Stay right with the physical-energetic experience of moving your focus, continuing slowly up your leg to your right knee. When you reach your right knee, stay right there. Allow yourself to maintain a singular concentration on your knee.

Now when you are ready, slowly move the focus of your attention from your right knee down your leg. Stay right with the experience of moving your focus, continuing slowly down your leg to your big toe. When you reach your big toe, maintain your focus right there.

After 1-2 minutes of focus, you can release your focus and open your eyes.

Questions to answer in your journal:

1. Were you able to maintain a clear connection with your body as you moved your focus of attention?
2. Did your focus jump around? For example, did you feel your toe and then lose connection with your foot, then feel your ankle? Journal about what you noticed in this regard.

Practice Support: If you found that your focus of attention seemed to jump around or that you blanked out at certain points of the exercise, take your time to learn how to stay connected with your body and your focus of attention. Slowing down and concentrating is essential. Initially it may be helpful for you to use your fingers to track the movement of your focus.

Recommended practice time is as many times as it takes to reach the desired result. Once you have accomplished this, please proceed to the Heart and Crown Meditation. There is no further need to continue with the warm-up.

Meditation

Close your eyes and focus your attention in the physical center of your heart chakra. *The center point lies midway between the surface of your chest and your spine.*

Hold your focus in your heart center. *Stay right there,* allowing yourself to relax into maintaining singular concentration. (Hold this focus for approximately 3-5 minutes.)

Now, very slowly move your focus from your heart up through the center of your upper chest – *staying right with the movement.* Continue to move your focus up through your neck and up through the top of your head to the center of your crown chakra. When you reach the center, *stay right there. (This center point will vary somewhat from person to person. Generally, it is positioned about 5-12 inches above the top of head. You will recognize it because it feels like a definite place.)*

Hold your focus in the center of your crown chakra. From time to time, notice how your body feels when you are focused here. (Hold this focus approximately 3-5 minutes.)

When you are ready, slowly move your focus of attention back down through the top of your head, staying right with the movement, down your neck and the center of your upper chest and into your heart chakra. Stay right there.

Hold your focus in the physical center of your heart chakra for 3-5 minutes. Notice how your body feels when you are focused here.

From this place of focus, look out from your heart. Open the *eyes in your heart* and look at the world around you. See your family, your friends, and your community; see the world with your heart. Hold this focus for as long as you wish.

When you feel complete, gently release your focus and open your eyes.

Questions to answer in your journal:
1. How do you feel energetically and emotionally?
2. Did you find the physical center of your heart chakra?
3. Did you stay with the movement of your focus?

4. Were you able to find the center of your crown chakra?

5. Were you able to see through the eyes of your heart? What did you feel and see?

6. Write about anything else you experienced.

Practice Support: This meditation can produce substantial energy gain. Immediately after you have answered all of the questions, lie down for 5-10 minutes while intending that your body absorb and use the energy you gained through the meditation. This is called *sponging.*

In general, quiet activities will always help you best absorb the energy and integrate your experience. When your schedule allows, give yourself one hour of quiet time following the meditation before re-entering your daily routine. This is especially important the first two or three times you practice it, because it will give you more opportunity to absorb energy.

When this time is up, check to see if you have any excess energy. Signs of excess energy include a slight headache, giddiness, or sudden hyperactivity. If necessary, release the excess through your tailbone into the Earth. As you have done before, you can do this simply by closing your eyes, focusing internally, and declaring that any excess energy go out your tailbone into the Earth. Remember to always include the word, "excess."

Read the Integration material any time **after** you have completed sponging and checked for excess energy.

Integration for this practice begins on page 113.

Recommended time schedule is 2 weeks – practicing a maximum of 1 time every other day, a minimum of 1 time per week.

VI.
The Prayer Exercise

Praying is an intentional, spiritual act. In prayer, you express gratitude, connect with your God, and/or request a benefit for others or yourself. Prayer is also a state of mind and heart – an integration of certain abilities: seeing through the eyes of the heart, being present, and maintaining a supportive, compassionate intention. Practicing The Prayer Exercise will strengthen your heart chakra and cultivate these abilities, helping to liberate your mind from judgment, control, and fear. As you maintain your focus during this exercise, healing energy will flow from the transcendent depth of your heart chakra without any exertion of your personal energies.

Exercise for self-healing

The purpose of this exercise is to bring healing attention to a part of yourself that is in need. To benefit from this exercise, you will want to identify a certain time in your life that was difficult for you. (The time can be last week or twenty-five years ago.) Choose a particular event or situation that took place at that time, and see yourself as you looked then. It is this part of self that you will aid in The Prayer Exercise.

Close your eyes and focus your attention in your heart chakra. Bring the part of yourself that you wish to help *in front of you* so that you can see, feel, or sense him or her.

Connect with this part of yourself through your heart chakra and let your hearts establish resonance. *Resonance will naturally occur as the two of you meet, heart to heart. Rely on your inner direction to accomplish this.*

Internally verbalize your intention to bring healing support to this part of yourself.

Be fully attentive and present with your other self by staying focused in your heart chakra. Open the eyes of your heart to see and feel this self. See this part of you without judging or labeling or trying to direct him or her.

If you find that you start to analyze, judge, or speak to your other self, place your hands palm side up on top of your knees, left hand on left knee, right hand on right knee. This is the mudra, a meditation position, for detachment. It will help you maintain receptivity and curb your tendencies to judge or direct what is happening. Hold the mudra until you feel receptive again. However, do not overuse the mudra, because using the mudra continually will change the intention of what you are doing.

You may find that this other part of you begins to speak to you or reveal his or her emotions. Allow this to happen. Hold the experience and be receptive to your other self. *Holding* means being the spiritual container for this process – giving it a safe place to unfold.

If a spontaneous dialogue begins between the two of you, continue to be receptive, respond as is natural, but do not direct the conversation. *If you find that you are being directive, use the mudra again.*

Continue The Prayer Exercise until you recognize a healing shift. This might be that you have gained new information from the other part of you. He or she may have released defenses or deeply held emotions. You might also notice that you feel peace and/or have gained new perspective about the past. Whatever form of healing takes place, proceed to complete the process by thanking your other self for being present and then releasing him or her. **If you can't complete the process because you are losing focus or because you realize additional prayer sessions are needed or desired,** commit to continuing this healing process in a day or two. Thank this part of you and let him or her go. Open your eyes when you are ready.

Questions to answer in your journal:

> 1. Did you feel like you were able to see and feel this part of yourself in a receptive way?
> 2. What did you learn about this part of you and this time in your life?
> 3. Do you feel complete or have you committed to continue to work with yourself?
> 4. Write all of your other feelings and thoughts about the process.

Practice Support: The benefit of this exercise is cumulative. It develops and stabilizes the heart chakra and brings insights into your relationship with yourself. After you have finished this exercise, it may be helpful to hold yourself in your heart as you do in the Self-Nurturing Meditation and let your compassion and understanding for this part of yourself deepen.

Integration for both versions of this practice begins on page 116.

Recommended time schedule is 1-2 weeks. In that time period feel free to practice this 2-3 times each week or as needed to complete your process. However, 1 time during the practice period is sufficient in terms of the course purpose.

Exercise for supporting others through absentee healing

Take a few moments to consider if you have a friend or family member who could use healing support and prayer at this time. You may call this person for direct permission to proceed or you may rely solely on your intuition. If, during the process, the other person disappears or rejects your intention (this feels palpable, like something has been pushed back to you), accept this as a sign that she or he does not want your assistance. Psychically and energetically excuse yourself and release your intention.

Now proceed according to the self-healing instructions, *except this time* feel yourself standing or sitting in front of the other person. *This is accomplished through intention.* Continue step by step through the entire process. *Remaining receptive and accepting is very important. You may feel challenged to let go of labels or judgments you have placed upon this person. Please use the mudra as necessary.*

Continue The Prayer Exercise until you have reached a completion. As in self-healing, you may commit to continue to work with this person at another time. Always thank the person and let her or him go before releasing your focus. Open your eyes when you are ready.

Questions to answer in your journal:

1. Were you able to remain receptive?
2. What did you learn about yourself?
3. What did you learn about the other person?
4. Were you able to see this individual in a new way?
5. Write about anything else you experienced.

Practice Support: The Prayer Exercise, more than any of the other practices, requires focus that does not strongly energize your body. Consequently, you can easily lose your concentration. If this was your experience, I suggest that you try doing this exercise with the other person physically present with you. He or she can sit across from you with eyes closed, and simply relax; then you can proceed through the steps of The Prayer Exercise. This person's presence in the room will help you feel more grounded and activate more energy in your heart chakra. Your ability to stay alert will improve. And if you do lose your focus, it will be easier to recover it. Remember to use the mudra for detachment as needed. Once you do the exercise in this manner a couple of times, you will find it much easier to practice alone.

If, during an absentee practice, you ever question whether or not you are being intrusive, rest assured that through energetic receptivity *you will know*. When you are able to be receptive, you will feel the other person accepting connection with you or pushing it back (as explained in the exercise). If the person is unwilling to participate, always fully respect her or his choice.

You do not need to practice this exercise for others often. However, it is important to understand how to do it, so you can use it when a specific need arises. If you are a professional clinician or practitioner, this exercise can be used with great success to support other work you are doing with your clients. Use the exercise as you have done here, or learn to use it with an eyes-open focus during sessions with your clients.

Recommended time schedule for practice is 1-2 weeks coinciding with the self-healing version of the exercise. Practice 1 time at a minimum.

VII.
Opening the Physical Channel

Before proceeding with this exercise, you may want to review the material on the physical channel in the Context.

Opening the Physical Channel strengthens your connection to the energetic core of your body and awakens the relationship between your first and seventh chakras. In this exercise you relax and align your body in order to intentionally receive ascending energy. As energy flows upward through you, your physical channel will open and, *if you stay present in your body,* you will gently and naturally enter a meditative state.

Exercise

Please proceed with the following three exercises practicing them one at time or in sequence. If you plan to complete all three, allow yourself 45-60 minutes the first time. The key to these exercises is to properly align your body, making small postural adjustments as needed. *Be patient with this part of the process. It is worth taking time for.* **You may answer the questions after each part of the exercise or upon completion of all three.**

Sitting

Seat yourself on the floor using a cushion or a rolled-up pillow to raise your pelvis higher than your knees. If you prefer to sit in a chair, make sure you use a pillow to lift your hips. *The height relationship between your pelvis and knees is particularly important in this exercise, so make sure you are positioned on the edge of the pillow or cushion. You could also use a meditation bench.*

Close your eyes and take two or three cleansing breaths – breathing in very slowly and gently through your nose and exhaling very slowly and gently out your mouth.

Tip your pelvis slightly, so that you can feel your perineum is almost flush with the floor or seat of your chair. Intend that your first chakra area open. *This is accomplished by totally relaxing the perineum area.*

When it is open, you will feel energy rise effortlessly into your body. *Please note that you do not have to make this happen. Relaxation and receptivity are the catalysts. When energy rises, you will likely feel a sexual surge and/or a sense of expansion or warmth in your pelvis.*

Relax your lower abdomen and let this energy rise through your pelvis. Now, gently and intentionally adjust your posture by straightening your lumbar area; then relax your stomach.

As your posture aligns, the energy will continue to rise upward along your physical channel. You will feel the energy move into your stomach, chest, throat, and head as it rises. Let the energy flow through the top of your head.

If you feel the energy stop moving, it is because your posture is not quite correct. Take a moment to subtly adjust your spine. Try slightly rocking your pelvis and/or straightening your lumbar vertebrae by lifting your chest. Notice if you have your head tipped backward or tilted downward. Adjust your head so that it is level. Tuck your chin in slightly.

When the energy flows through the top of your crown chakra, you will feel as though your body is floating upward from the foundation of your pelvis. You may also feel as though someone is gently pulling you upward from the top of your head. Allow yourself to enjoy this for as long as you wish.

When you feel ready, gently release your focus and open your eyes.

Please note: If you do not wish to continue on to the standing position of the exercise at this time, wait 10 minutes, then close your eyes and internally verbalize your intention that your ascending and descending energies balance.

Opening the Physical Channel does not usually cause excess energy gain but might result in a "too open" feeling. In this case, you may use the following breathing exercise.

As you inhale, expand your auric field slightly. As you exhale, contract your aura to bring it closer to your body 3-4 inches. *Use intention to accomplish this.* Repeat 2-3 times. This technique is very grounding and balancing and can be used any time you feel scattered, ungrounded, or weakened physically.

If you bring your aura too close to your body, you will experience pressure against your arms, head, and/or chest. If this happens, simply expand your auric field 3-4 inches as necessary.

Questions to answer in your journal:

    1. How does your body feel physically and energetically?
    2. Was your mind quiet during the exercise?
    3. Did you feel a lifting sensation through your spine?
    4. Did you feel yourself move into a meditative state?
    5. How do you feel emotionally and mentally?
    6. Write about anything else you experienced.

Practice Support: If you had any trouble with your postural alignment, be confident that the trouble will lessen with time. You will soon adjust to having an open physical channel, and it will happen without effort. Being able to open the physical channel will help you in all your meditations since it facilitates sitting comfortably for longer periods. Reading the Integration material will be helpful at any time after you answer the questions for each of the three phases of this exercise.

Integration for all three versions of this practice begins on page 120.

Recommended time schedule is 2 weeks – practicing 1 time every other day for a week; then, every day if you wish. You may practice the exercise fewer times during this period if you prefer, but I would not recommend more times. It is also important to try the other two methods of Opening the Physical Channel. Thereafter you may wish to use all three during your practice period or just focus on your favorite.

Standing

Stand with your feet about shoulder width apart. Open the soles of your feet to the Earth by relaxing the area below the arch of your foot. Allow energy to rise upward. As you feel the energy rise into your feet, relax your knees to allow the energy to rise upward into your legs. Now, open the first chakra area. *Slightly bending your knees and slightly tucking in your pelvis will help you align your posture and allow the energy to continue to rise into your body. The main key to facilitating the standing position is to keep the soles of the feet open and the first chakra relaxed.*

When you feel energy enter your pelvis, continue to adjust your posture to find the correct alignment. Energy will move upward through your body and eventually through the top of your head just as in the sitting position. *The solar plexus area can be difficult to align. As in the sitting posture, keeping your lumbar area straight will help you find the correct position. Sometimes lowering your chin slightly will also help. Relaxing your shoulders may be necessary.*

When the energy has risen through your entire body and out the top of your head, you will feel your body floating upward from the foundation of your feet. After a few minutes in this position, release your focus and open your eyes.

If you are not continuing on to the next exercise, within about 10 minutes verbalize your intention that your ascending and descending energies balance.

Practice Support: If you find that this standing posture is difficult, practice the exercise lying down. After practicing it this way a few times, you will likely find it easier to do the standing exercise. When lying down, you continue to use your feet as the entrance point for ascending energy.

Walking

This exercise is wonderful to practice outside, especially in a large park, in the mountains, or in the desert. You may, of course, practice it inside as well.

First open your physical channel in the standing posture. When you feel yourself floating from the foundation of your feet, open your eyes slightly and begin to walk very slowly. *The key to fulfilling this exercise is to keep the soles of your feet open and walk slowly enough at the beginning to keep your focus.*

As you continue to move, you may choose to quicken your pace a little, walking more naturally. Continue as long as you wish with your eyes now fully open. When you are ready to stop, stand still for a couple of minutes before releasing your focus.

Practice Support: Take your time during the slow part of the walking process. This initial connection is important. As you begin to pick up speed, check in occasionally with the soles of your feet. You will notice that your feet feel soft and very alive.

You will probably fully absorb the energy gained while walking. Likewise, your descending energy will usually balance automatically. However, if you wish, wait about 20 minutes after completing the exercise and verbalize your intention that your ascending and descending energies balance.

VIII.
Reference Point Meditation

Your soul center, located deep in your heart chakra, is the spiritual mind of your body and consciousness. Through it you *see* and ultimately assimilate life experience. To sustain relationship with your deep heart is to be able to accept and digest life in the context of spiritual identity and selfhood. The soul center, or reference point, offers you a sanctuary for inner peace.

Exercise

Close your eyes and focus your attention in the physical center of your heart chakra.

Focus deeper and deeper in your heart chakra as though you were sinking into it. *It is important to feel this physically; you are moving toward, but not to, your spine.*

Continue with this focus until you are able to find the place in your heart chakra that feels like an opening from which energy is flowing forward. This is your reference point. *Take your time finding the reference point. Reaching it may mean entering a deeper space than you might have imagined.*

While focused in your reference point, allow yourself to feel the energy as it flows forward and fills your entire body. *The flow of energy can feel subtle and somewhat rhythmical. Do not make it happen, simply be aware of it. While you are sensing this, keep your focus in your reference point as well.*

When the energy has filled your body, notice it moving beyond your body into your auric field. Be attentive to the energy as it fills your auric field.

Once the aura is full, be aware of the circulation of this energy as it flows back into your body. Receive it. *Stay very present in your body and in your reference point. Remain attentive to the circulation of energy for 4-10 minutes; longer is fine too.*

When you are ready, gently release your focus and open your eyes.

Questions to answer in your journal:

1. How do you feel?
2. Were you able to find your reference point? Were you able to maintain focus in your reference point during the meditation?

3. Were you able to feel the circulation of energy?

4. Write about anything else you experienced.

Practice Support: The key to this meditation is reaching your reference point. If you found this difficult, try again, and remember to focus your attention physically in your heart chakra. To find this physical place, you may want to first take a deep, full breath. You will feel a channel open in your chest. Go to the place within that channel *in your heart chakra*. From this spot begin moving back to your reference point.

When you can maintain the physical focus and move it inward toward your spine, you will discover the place where energy is flowing into your heart. This sensation can feel very subtle. You may not notice it in a direct way, but instead, feel an opening in your back or recognize an immediate sense of internal quiet.

The reference point is the gateway to transcendent energy. It is the point of interface where the body meets the energy of the soul. As you attempt to find it, you may feel that you are going very, very deep – and keeping your focus once you find it may require a new level of concentration. However, once you become familiar with it, you will find your reference point not subtle at all. Rather, it becomes an easily accessible destination, your sanctuary of stillness and peace.

Read the Integration material whenever you wish for additional support with this meditation.

Integration for this practice begins on page 123.

Recommended time schedule for the Reference Point Meditation is 1–2 weeks. You may practice it daily or less often. However, it is helpful to have at least 3 successful experiences with this meditation before going on to the next one.

IX.
Soul Force Meditation

As much as you are a physical being, you are a nonphysical one. You are energy, will, and consciousness. Your energy system is an instrument of this totality, embodying your physical, personal, and transcendent energies and reflecting your overall awareness.

Throughout the energetic practices of this course work, you have relied on your energy system to bring you to new experiences and varied states of consciousness. The Soul Force Meditation completes the series by guiding you to use the energetic gateway of the reference point to bring your soul's vital energy, *the soul force,* into your body.

You began this course by coming to your heart and you complete it in the same way. Open your heart inwardly to yourself and welcome the subtle energy of your soul force into your body. *Know yourself.*

Meditation

Practice this meditation in a room where you can remain solely by yourself. It is not appropriate to work with your soul force around other people. Further information about this is found in the Integration section.

Close your eyes and take two or three gentle cleansing breaths, inhaling very slowly and gently through your nose and exhaling very slowly and gently out your mouth.

Now, focus in your reference point. *Take your time to make a strong connection.*

When you are ready, ask your soul force to come through your reference point. *You may feel your soul force as a strong or subtle shift in your energy. You may feel physical warmth or experience a sense of expansion or lightness. Each person's soul force is different, bearing its own tempo and vibratory rate.*

Allow your soul force energy to fill your heart chakra and your body. *You do this through intention and/or an internal affirmation.*

When your body is full, lift your hands and allow your soul force to flow out (channel) through your hands and into the room. *Hold your hands up to the side of your body at chest height and face your palms forward into the room. Do not let your hands block the torso of your body.*

Continue channeling your soul force until you wish to stop. *An ideal length of time is 10 minutes. Initially this may feel very long. However, it is important to stay with it long enough to gain confidence with the meditation.*

When you feel ready to stop, close the outflow of soul force in the palms of your hands. *You can do this by intention alone or by intention and closing your fingers over your palms.*

You can then release your focus and open your eyes.

Questions to answer in your journal:

1. How do you feel?
2. Were you able to feel your soul force?
3. Were you able to feel the outflow stop? If not, close your eyes and close the outflow again.
4. Write about anything else you experienced.

Practice Support: Your soul force can seem very subtle in contrast to the energy you have activated in other practices. Your soul force is a purely transcendent energy and may not cause a strong change in your body. However, if you remain alert during the meditation, you will notice that your soul force brings a frequency change throughout your overall energy system, especially in your heart chakra. Take time to discern the gentle shifts that accompany your soul force and notice how your mental and emotional experiences alter.

If you had any difficulty sustaining your focus throughout this meditation, it probably is due to either a lack of confidence or your inability to stay deep in your heart chakra. Confidence will come over time and through practice. However, maintaining focus in your reference point will require intention on your part. You can reinforce connection with your deep heart often during the meditation by simply *pushing back into the reference point*. Once you are reconnected, your soul force energy will come forth. Further information within the Integration material will help you with these challenges.

Please note: Sometimes connecting with your soul force can be unwittingly compromised by your close connection to spirit guides. If you strongly rely on your guides or guardians to help you in your daily life, you can become quite merged with them energetically. Just prior to practicing this meditation, ask your guides to temporarily step away from you energetically. This will give you a chance to recognize your soul force, which is also a source of help in your life. Rest assured that the request you make to your guides will be understood and will not result in any weakening of relationship with them.

I recommend that you read the corresponding Integration section as soon as you are ready, even after the first practice.

Integration for this practice begins on page 124.

Recommended schedule is 2 weeks – no more than once per day. After you have finished the Integration material, please read the Epilogue. It will give you guidelines for how to most naturally continue to use the meditations.

Part III

Integration

SELF-HEALING IS REALIZED THROUGH THE ACTS, THOUGHTS, INTENTIONS, AND SPOKEN WORDS OF DAILY LIFE.

ALL LEARNING, ESPECIALLY LEARNING focused on internal experience, requires assimilation and practical application to become a true resource. The process of digesting and applying what you are now discovering constitutes integration work. Taking time with integration will enrich your relationship with the practices, helping you to understand their influences and discover how to best use them in your life.

The information in this section of the book incorporates direct feedback from students along with my own teaching intent. This material outlines the course purpose, the common benefits and applications, the common challenges, and the energetic influences of each practice. The best way to use the Integration is to first, upon completing each exercise, answer the list of questions that follow the practice. Once you have used the exercise a second time, you have adequate personal experience to reference and can proceed with the Integration.

Self-Nurturing Meditation

Course Purpose: The Self-Nurturing Meditation focuses on developing a compassionate and responsive relationship with yourself. It asks you to connect with your heart and draw your focus and nurturing inward. This meditation is a foundational practice of self-care.

As you hold yourself in your heart and receive your own love and compassion, you open and strengthen your heart chakra. The inflowing energy (love), as well as the affirmations, loosens the hold of self-negating attitudes and beliefs that deplete or block your heart chakra. Supporting your heart in this way will help you experience and express the true nature of this chakra – discernment, unconditional love, compassion for self and others, and spiritual resolution of all life experiences.

Common Benefits and Applications: The first positive influence of this meditation is that it confronts the false belief that self-love is selfish. *Fear of being selfish* can be a powerful belief, often rooted in religious and/or familial conditioning. Fear of being selfish can divert you from your personal desires, proper use of will, and true motivations in life. It can persuade you to place the needs and pleasure of others above those of self. In some cases, such beliefs can lead to extreme attitudes of self-denial or self-negation. Energetic blockage, contraction, or congestion around the chest (heart chakra) and/or stomach area (third chakra) can result.

If you carry any of these beliefs and stresses, the Self-Nurturing Meditation will be of great benefit to you. The energetic action of holding yourself in your heart and receiving your own love will counteract your conditioning and self-negating beliefs. Over time as you practice this meditation, a new resonance of self-valuing will develop within you. Internally, you will begin to grow new faculties of discernment and choice. Soon you will *know* the difference between self-nurturing attitudes and behaviors and self-negating ones.

To use the Self-Nurturing Meditation as a healing tool, I recommend that you practice it on a regular basis – either daily or every other day. If your stress and conditioning are extreme, I also recommend that you seek the help of a qualified therapist or healer to help you uncover and release the causal factors. I suggest that you continue to use this meditation as a complementary, therapeutic tool. Holding yourself in your heart and inflowing energy will enhance all other healing you experience and integrate it into your body. Making this physical connection is essential to deepen and ground what you are discovering.

Use the Self-Nurturing Meditation anytime you are experiencing a disconnection from or a weakening of self. Disconnection or weakening can be chronic or acute. Chronic challenges can come from childhood or adult-age abuse or neglect *or* chronic alcohol or drug abuse. Recovering from any of these experiences is a multilevel process that ultimately centers on reclaiming and retrieving self. Connection with your heart and your body is pivotal. This meditation along with practices II, III, and IV will support you in this process.

Sudden, acute disconnection from or weakening of self can occur when you work or live as a caregiver *or* anytime you overextend yourself. The affirmations and energy work of the Self-Nurturing Meditation refresh the heart and allow self to once again take a central position. Practicing this meditation on a regular basis helps you avoid the extremes of exhaustion and resentment that

Self as center

esp. when caring for others.

94

may build up without you even realizing it. If you are unable to inflow energy using the Self-Nurturing Meditation, remember to practice Hands Over Heart.

Common Challenges: If you find that this meditation repeatedly challenges you, I suggest that you read it again line by line, exploring the meaning of each affirmation. You may find that you need to replace certain words to make the meditation more truthful and relevant to you. Or, you may discover that you have conflicting beliefs in regard to one or all of the affirmations. In this case, I recommend that you journal about the specific statements you do not agree with or process them with a friend.

Here are three examples of how to process common challenges with the affirmations in this meditation.

1. If you find self-forgiveness difficult, examine your past actions, behaviors, or interchanges with others that you deem unforgivable. Now think about and identify your level of understanding at the time of each occurrence. Acknowledge your motivations. You can then determine what you actually *knew* and *did not know* at the time. Write your responses in your journal; then answer the following questions.

How would you feel about another person who had the same understanding and motivation as you did and acted similarly? Would you feel compassion for him or her? Could you forgive this person and release him or her from the limitation of that experience? If you answer "yes," will you then forgive yourself?

Self-forgiveness is an essential step in both energetic and spiritual well-being. It releases the energy and the emotion held in the past and allows you to evolve into the present. Your potential for further growth and learning is then truly realizable.

2. During the meditation, if you are unwilling or unable to hear what you need, exploring your beliefs and conditioning concerning

need will be helpful. You can use the following questions as a guide.

Do you consider need to be an issue of physical survival only? Are you willing to consider need in terms of emotional, psychological, and spiritual survival as well? Do you equate need with neediness?

Neediness usually reflects a belief or feeling that one is not powerful enough or adequate to address one's own needs. If you feel unable to effectively address your needs, take the time to review your family history as elicited by the following questions.

How were needs expressed in your family? How did your family respond to the needs of one another? Were needs looked upon as a sign of weakness? Do you feel ashamed of your needs? On a scale of 1 to 10, how empowered do you feel to address and meet your own needs?

By answering these questions and identifying your relationship to and beliefs around *need,* you will begin to step beyond your conditioning. To establish new ideas and behaviors, you will want to continue, perhaps on a daily basis, to explore and name what you need.

Some needs are immediate, focusing on the day-to-day, hour-to-hour conditions. Some needs reflect long-term issues such as relationships, employment, lifestyle, etc. To truly appreciate your needs, consider how *needs* are the signposts of your changing requirements for well-being, survival, personal integrity, and spiritual unfolding. Committing to meet your own needs is an act of self-nurturing and compassion that allows you to thrive rather than merely survive in life.

If you have spent years denying or ignoring your needs, it may take a little time to awaken the *need voice* within you. However, committing yourself to this discovery will be life changing. In your exploration of need, do not analyze if your need is real or merely a *want.* Just listen to your heart and body and *do not judge.* Instead be curious, ask yourself why the need or want is important to you. Your answers will inform you and *reveal* you.

Do not judge need

3. Some students feel unclear about the affirmation that states that they are responsible for being a creative force in their own lives. It is very important for you – for everyone – to establish a baseline understanding and philosophy about personal power in life. This understanding can be based on a perspective that *life is chosen and not a design of fate*. It may be founded on an attitude that *no matter what happens in your life, you will handle it and meet the challenge.* The particular belief is not what is important. What is important is that you have a way to gather your resources, use your will, and be accountable to yourself. The following questions may help you recognize your own beliefs in this area.

What is your personal belief about your own power in this life? How do you survive hard times? What motivates you to overcome challenges? Do you create the life you want? If not, what stops you? Once you clarify your own parameters for self-empowerment, reword the affirmation in the exact way that reflects your truth on this matter.

Energetic Influence: Energetically, this meditation is the first step in exercising your *receiving muscle*. The inflow of love equals the inflow of energy. As energy enters your heart chakra, your entire energy system begins to replenish. This first stage of energetic strengthening helps you open the pathway to the soul center within your heart chakra.

Hands Over Heart

The ability to receive energy is a key function of your energy system and an essential factor in your health. Receiving energy allows you to restore the energy you use and build reserves that sustain your aura, chakras, physical channel, and meridians. On the consciousness level, receiving and retaining energy help maintain mental clarity, effective use of will, emotional balance, and a greater connection with self.

If the Self-Nurturing Meditation challenges you and you are unable to receive love – energy – into your heart, there may be several causes. The inability to receive energy can either be an acute or chronic condition. Acute stress can come from many sources – an argument with a loved one, extreme fatigue, loss of someone close to you, or self-criticism. Under any of these conditions, you may outflow energy at a rapid rate, or conversely, contract into a state of energetic paralysis. Your heart chakra will tighten or close. The Hands Over Heart exercise quickly and gently restores your ability to take in energy.

Placing your hand(s) over your heart chakra can be done anywhere you can gather a few moments for yourself. Your hands give you contact with your body, energy system, and self. They give you physical protection and support. Energetically, your hands produce a gentle current of energy that will flow into your heart chakra. When you first begin to practice this exercise, you may not be able to feel the energy itself. However, as the energy begins to flow into the heart, you may notice that you take a deep breath or drop your shoulders. These are signs that you are receiving and that circulation of energy is reactivated.

Chronic stress that limits receptivity is always the result of trauma (which can include any form of abuse, neglect, life-negating circumstances, illness, or accidents), belief structure, and/or conditioning. In these cases, vulnerability and openness are considered a threat or a negative in some way. When receptivity has become a threatening experience, small, gentle steps toward healing are best.

If you suffer from chronic stress, placing your hands over your heart is a way to aid yourself. You may wish to begin by using the Hands Over Heart Exercise in the evening before retiring. (It is fine if you fall asleep during the exercise.) When you are ready to expand your practice time, using this exercise during the day will help you inflow restorative energy. Little by little receiving energy will become a comforting rather than vulnerable experience.

Inflow Exercise

Course Purpose: Your vital energy is a personal resource. To understand how to best maintain this resource, you need to recognize how you are using it and how you may be losing it. You must also learn how to retrieve your energy and how to conserve it. The Inflow Exercise offers you a direct way to replenish your energy and encourages you to retain it.

Common Benefits and Applications: In the most practical of all applications, the Inflow Exercise can be used as part of your daily self-maintenance routine. When used after work or at the end of your day, you can gather your energy and regain energetic, physical, and emotional balance. Inflowing your energy nourishes and replenishes your nervous system as well as your adrenals. This exercise can be done so easily and in such little time that you might try replacing your afternoon coffee break with the Inflow.

The Inflow can also be used to directly retrieve your energy from a specific situation or person. For instance, if you argue or strongly disagree with someone, you exert energy. If the interchange is unresolved, you can feel frustrated or experience a sense of loss. Under these circumstances, you will not naturally regain the energy you have expended.

When you lose energy to someone, you will be signaled in one or both of the following ways. First, you will feel depleted, not simply tired; you are going to feel drained. Second, you may find yourself replaying an interaction over and over again in your mind. This is a sign that you are trying to reconnect with *your* energy. You are focusing on the event *where your energy has been left*. Practicing the Inflow Exercise will retrieve your energy. It will also reduce your angst about the situation and the other person(s) involved.

Simply practice the Inflow Exercise, as you normally would, except this time call your energy back from the particular situation and person(s). Upon the return of your energy, your understanding

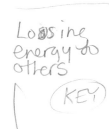

General Inflow or Inflow from Situation or Person

Loosing energy to others (KEY)

of the experience will be clearer. If you need to re-engage, you can do so with more self-awareness and perspective. Over time you will be able to learn how to better manage an argument or discussion – tempering your vigor, attachment, and outflow of energy while still supporting your point of view.

Using the Inflow Exercise is easy; however, remembering to or being willing to use it may be a challenge. It is a great freedom and a great responsibility to know that you alone have the choice to call your energy back. Making or refusing to make the choice constitutes an act of will on your part. *Empower yourself.*

This exercise can also help if you are recently divorced or if you have lost someone through death. In both cases, your grieving process needs to be respected and allowed to fulfill itself. However, if you find that you are struggling to maintain emotional balance, practice the Inflow from time to time. Doing so will reduce your sense of loss and help you move forward in your life. In this application, call your energy directly back from the person for whom you are grieving. Then send back any energy you carry that belongs to this person. *Remember, do not send back the other's energy until after retrieving your own.*

If a separation, divorce, or breakup becomes toxic or entangled, use the Inflow Exercise often, followed by Practice III, Clearing and Sealing the Auric Field. Recovering and protecting your energy by using these exercises will keep your mind and emotions in balance.

Please note: The Inflow Exercise can be used to retrieve energy from any situation or relationship in the past that you feel is unresolved or incomplete. Practice it to help heal a traumatic or challenging event by calling back *your energy* from the specific circumstance you wish to complete. If you want to address a past relationship, follow directions described previously. If you feel a need to repeat this process in regard to a particular situation or relationship, allow 5 to 7 days between practice times, so that you can integrate.

Common Challenges: When students find this practice to be a challenge, it is primarily because receiving, in general, is uncomfortable for them. If you find this to be the case for you, support your body by placing your hand(s) over your heart during the Inflow. It is important to be patient in this process. If you are not used to receiving, you will have built up certain armor – patterns of tension and tightness in your body – that will need to soften. Regular focus and time given to the Self-Nurturing Meditation, the Hands Over Heart exercise, and the Inflow will bring transformational results, and eventually receiving energy will feel natural.

Energetic Influence: Building the health of your energy system depends on your ability to maintain a reserve of energy. The Inflow Exercise builds your *receiving muscle*. It also recovers energy that you exert. Regular Inflow practice will help you develop healthy energy habits that will lead to your retaining more energy.

Clearing and Sealing the Auric Field

Course Purpose: The aura energetically reflects who you are. It also contains who you are by creating an energetic environment and boundary around your body. Maintaining the strength of the auric field is essential to maintaining your overall health and sense of self.

Clearing and Sealing the Auric Field offers a direct means by which you can protect and strengthen the vital energy of your aura. It teaches you to recognize who and what you allow to use your energy. Your energy field exists to sustain *you*. Others have their own energy fields that likewise sustain them. Practicing this exercise clarifies these boundaries.

Common Benefits and Applications: Clearing and Sealing the Auric Field will help you transform specific beliefs, conditioning, and behaviors that create weak boundaries. It will also promote the healing of chronically weak or damaged boundaries. Practice this meditation if you have suffered physical, emotional, sexual, and/or psychological abuse or you are working to end addiction to alcohol or drugs. In all of these situations, your boundaries have been compromised. Clearing and Sealing the Auric Field will reestablish boundaries and help you clear away the unwanted intrusions from others.

Chronically weak, damaged, or diffuse energetic boundaries create and reinforce a disconnection from self. *Bringing boundaries into focus means bringing self into focus.* Learning to recognize self – identifying your emotions, needs, responsibilities, desires, etc. – takes time. If you have chronic conditions to heal, I recommend that you do complementary work with a qualified healer or therapist to further address emotional and psychological issues. If your body has become weakened because of substance abuse or neglect of self, I would also recommend that you see a doctor of traditional Chinese medicine or a naturopathic physician. Continue to practice Clearing and Sealing the Auric Field, preferably on a daily basis, over an extended period of time.

Clearing and Sealing the Auric Field can also be used to clear away the unwanted influences of others, releasing you from their projections, demands, and other forms of mental or emotional coercion. Whether these influences have been intentionally thrust upon you or are merely the result of another's immaturity and your own naiveté, they can have disruptive results. Your personal values, goals, dreams, and health can be compromised. I typically suggest this exercise for students and clients who no longer recognize their own personal goals or who have recently left a demanding or destructive relationship, organization, or job.

Re-identification with oneself is a joy and fosters productivity. Personal creativity, dreams, and goals generate energy. Consider using Clearing and Sealing the Auric Field to stimulate your creative process and strengthen your life focus. Like the Inflow Exercise, you can also use this exercise to replenish yourself.

You can practice it more frequently after completing a long-term project or giving a great deal of energy to another person. I have also seen Clearing and Sealing the Auric Field heal anger and resentment. A past student, who is a mother and elementary school teacher, was growing increasingly impatient, but did not realize that her energetic boundaries were severely compromised. Using this practice on a regular basis restored her sense of self, healed escalating stress, and transformed her relationships with *all* of her children.

Common Challenges: Many students find that this practice challenges their beliefs about caring for others. They find it difficult to set people they love outside their auric boundary. They feel concerned that energetically separating from people they are close to will cause disconnection. Some students believe that they *must* keep other people in the auric field in order to sustain the well-being of those persons.

If you have similar beliefs, do not fear that setting another person outside your auric field will disconnect you or place someone or something at risk. A well-defined boundary simply allows you and the other individual to function as whole people with healthy, self-referencing capabilities. Practicing this meditation can remind you that everyone has an aura and has boundaries, *including* small children and individuals who are ill or in need. It is important to understand and respect the wholeness of others even though you are protecting them or serving their need for care.

When a situation, project, or challenge demands your energy, be aware that holding the specific concern too close can prevent that endeavor from flourishing or garnering outside support. If you attach yourself to it out of a sense of responsibility, others will not be attracted to step forward to contribute. Situations and projects, like people, are their own entities. Although they do not possess boundaries as such, they do possess energy. Letting a situation or project exist as separate from you will let it evolve as it should *and do so without draining you.*

Other challenges with this practice come from its strengthening effects. As a result of establishing clearer boundaries, students find that they suddenly act more independently. Some welcome this change. For others, this behavior feels unnatural and they question its value. If this is your experience, you may want to explore your own history with unclear boundaries. Write in your journal about past experiences involving *asserting or not asserting your will, taking care of others, and knowing or not knowing what you want. Take time to acknowledge what unclear boundaries have cost you.* After completing this writing, you will realize why having stronger boundaries is essential and how it reflects your healthy evolution.

If you have formed relationships based on your having unclear boundaries and not thinking or acting in your own best interests, your new attitudes and behaviors may upset others. Give your family and friends time to adapt. Consider using a mediation model for communicating with them if conflicts or hurt feelings arise. Taking time to hear the needs and wishes of one another and identify common ground issues will open a dialogue and help valued relationships evolve. Remember common ground concerns can be better communication or mutual love and respect.

If, however, you discover that certain individuals are unwilling to experiment and grow along with you, you can learn to maintain your boundaries without their approval and incorporate "No" into your vocabulary. Your clarity will allow others to recalibrate the relationship in their own way.

Energetic Influence: The aura is a substantial energy resource. It directly interfaces with the chakras and the entrance points of the meridians and influences both. This practice strengthens your energy and your energy system by improving and protecting the integrity of the aura.

Chakra Clearing and Balancing

Course Purpose: Chakra work represents a substantial section of this course because your chakras are major indicators of the immediate condition of your consciousness and body. Interaction with the chakras through the use of energy, emotional or psychological processing, and spiritual intention brings beneficial results almost instantaneously. Thus, understanding the chakras – their governing issues *and* how to work with them – is essential to maintaining and strengthening the energy system.

Common Benefits and Applications: One of the greatest benefits of chakra work is that through it you are able to develop a direct line of communication with your body and better facilitate physical healing. Students typically use chakra work whenever they feel any discomfort near a specific chakra area. I have seen sore throats, mild digestive maladies, localized infections, and vertebrae misalignments quickly helped by chakra work. In many cases, chakra work alone completely cleared the challenge. In very serious or chronic diseases and conditions like pneumonia, heart problems, migraines, ulcers, and asthma, chakra work offers energetic renewal that will support other healing treatments. It will also bring the corresponding consciousness issues to the surface and promote their clearing.

As consciousness centers, chakras reveal the deepest truths of the psyche, often exposing *what the mind denies*. Because chakra work taps information in its energetic form, it is not dependent on the mind's cooperation for results. Consequently, chakra work is highly effective. Dialoguing with chakras or accurately reading their energies will *always* result in energetic movement and some degree of healing. Students have successfully used chakra work to address a variety of life issues and experiences including poor self-esteem, inability to forgive oneself, unresolved trauma, anger, or rage, and depression. Chakra work can be the sole healing method used or it can complement another modality.

In the context of your soul's evolution, your chakras are powerful allies and facilitators. Not only do chakras record current lifetime experiences, they carry over past life information to be utilized or resolved in the present. Connecting with your chakras on a regular basis through the Revitalization Exercises or Chakra Phrases will help you keep in contact with this energetic information and history. And then when you need it, when something of a karmic nature is trying to surface and resolve, you will be able to easily access it and use it for your own healing.

Common Challenges: When students are first introduced to the chakras, they often express a feeling of being overwhelmed. They feel suddenly and *completely* confronted with the totality of who they are. Yet, there is a more comforting way to look at it. Your consciousness, energy, and body are alive; they are fluid, changing, growing. Understanding and working with the chakra system is simply the best way to establish deep, immediate, and ongoing communication with self.

The greatest challenge of the chakra work is that it requires us to acknowledge who we are and what we feel. Most of us have times of challenge in our lives – times of hurt, loss, or great struggle. We develop ways to cope with and survive these experiences. However, we may not be fully able to resolve them. We may instead choose to deny them, hide from our feelings, and/or close ourselves to painful areas of life. Chakra work will uncover and awaken what remains undigested from those experiences. In other words, *chakra work initiates and promotes recovery.*

Even though the rewards of chakra work are great, there may be conditions or situations that you do not feel ready to deal with. If this is your experience, I want to reassure you that you can choose to leave some needed work *on the shelf.* You may instead work with other issues and chakras that you feel ready to handle. You can always decide later to focus on the more difficult and challenging situations, taking them off the shelf.

Here is a closer look at three specific chakras that consistently challenge students:

1. The **second chakra** concerns itself primarily with issues of power, self-containment, nurturing, and deep connection with others. Students of both sexes can find their second chakras chronically stressed. However, women often embody one consistent conflict. Many women will describe how much of their energy and efforts go to caring for their families and securing a relationship with their partner. These same women say that they feel weak-willed, unfulfilled, and lacking in personal power.

The second chakra activities of caring for a family and focusing on relationship emphasize *merging and nurturing*. Energetically these activities can create an outflow of energy, which can lead to minor or extreme depletion. Self-containment is also governed by the second chakra. Containment refers to the ability to hold and conserve one's energy as a source of personal power and strength. Containment requires clear boundaries and balances outflow.

If you find that you outflow too much energy and lose balance in the second chakra, I recommend that you try the following exercise:

1. Close your eyes and focus your attention in your second chakra.
2. Internally direct your energy to flow from the center of the second chakra upward to your heart chakra.
3. Hold this focus for 5-10 minutes.
4. When you are ready, release your focus and open your eyes.

During this exercise did you feel a physical sense of inner strength and containment? If you did, keep practicing this exercise. If you did not feel it, *keep practicing this exercise.* This exercise, along with thoughtful self-examination, will help you correct second chakra imbalances.

It is important to remember that the second chakra governs a set of complex issues – many that involve sexual roles and identities. Therefore, expression of second chakra issues varies in context from culture to culture, religion to religion, and family to family. It will be helpful for you to consider these external influences as you work with your second chakra.

2. The **third chakra** is another chakra that challenges many students. The third chakra focuses on issues of individuation, self-awareness, and enjoyment of and participation in life. A strong and healthy third chakra reflects an attitude of self-acceptance and self-advocacy. The third chakra affirms, "I am a self."

When describing a healthy third chakra, I often refer to it as having the persona of a happy five-year-old. Five-year-olds strongly identify with what they want and eagerly represent it. Their innocent verbalization of ideas, observations, and feelings is delightfully uncensored and lacks self-criticism and attachment. Vitality, natural confidence, and joy for life exude from them.

As we mature, we adjust the five-year-old persona in favor of more appropriate sensibilities and responsibilities. However natural and beneficial this maturing process seems, it can sharply compromise our fulfillment of third chakra issues. Symptoms of a diminished third chakra can include denying or overriding one's emotions, being reasonable *all the time*, withdrawing from enjoyable activities, loss of self-referencing skills, poor digestion, migraine headaches (third chakra generally is the causal level), and any illnesses centered in the third chakra area.

If you experience low-grade or occasional acute stress in your third chakra, I recommend that you take time to rediscover your emotions, wants, and needs. Daily journaling in which you describe the events of your day and openly and honestly voice your accompanying emotions and thoughts will help restore your third chakra. On paper or with a friend, allow yourself to say, *to confess*, what you want and need. If your wants and needs seem unrealistic, irresponsible, overwhelming, etc., *do not stop*, continue to reveal them.

Your wants and needs are meaningful to different parts of you, and discovering their relevance is essential to fully understanding and *representing* who you are. When you identify your want or need, find out why it is important by asking yourself what fulfilling that want or need will give you. When you hear the answer, *validate it* – do not assess it. In doing so, your third chakra energy will improve and you will lay the foundation for clearer self-advocating action and decision making.

After reading the above material, you may recognize that your third chakra imbalances are not occasional, they are chronic. Longstanding third chakra stress most often reflects core childhood or adult experiences of neglect, restriction, and/or abuse or family dynamics that negated third chakra issues.

When a child's wants, needs, and feelings are denied or invalidated and/or when a child is physically, psychologically, and/or emotionally abused, her or his blossoming ego is not able to develop properly. The happy five-year-old persona of the third chakra may never be born or may psychically leave at a very young age. The key strengths and attributes of this chakra likewise do not manifest. When an adult experiences abuse, neglect or negation, her or his responses are similar; the third chakra will shut down or be severely psychically damaged.

Extreme third chakra damage can result in a complete denial or an overcompensation of the third chakra domain. Denial of this chakra can lead to many life-negating behaviors and choices such as sacrifice of self and personal abilities, drug or alcohol abuse, eating disorders, and repeated co-dependent or abusive relationships. Overcompensation for a damaged third chakra may manifest as drug or alcohol abuse, workaholic behavior, abusiveness toward self or others, or extreme self-centeredness and defensiveness. Often a person will engage in both denial and overcompensation.

If you have experienced childhood or adult abuse and have suppression or other damage in the third chakra, you will benefit from a long-term process of healing. Depending on your personal history, your process may extend over months, several years, or a great part of your life. If this is your experience, I want to assure you that healing can still occur. I would, however, advise you to find a specialized therapist or healer skilled at working with life situations like your own. Continued work with chakra revitalization, phrases, and journaling about feelings, wants, and needs will complement these efforts.

Whenever you are challenged with acute or chronic stress from the third chakra, focusing on the heart chakra will often bring relief. The heart chakra supports connection with self through acceptance, unconditional love, and release. You will find that doing energy work in the fourth chakra or a meditation such as the Self-Nurturing Meditation will help you clear, soothe, and heal the third chakra.

3. The **fifth chakra** represents and reflects issues of self-expression, communication, creativity, and the choice *to be.* Some students recognize fifth chakra stress because they have chronic sore throats and have difficulty expressing their feelings and ideas. Others notice that they want to or *do* control other people. These students describe forceful conversations in which they refuse to listen to another's perspectives or ideas and try to bend others to their own will. All of these fifth chakra issues can be helped through processing and confronting personal beliefs and conditioning. However, there is also an energetic approach that is effective and quickly facilitates balancing of the fifth chakra. To work with this method, it helps to understand the energetic dynamics of the throat.

The throat is a center where energy from the Infinite directly enters the body. This interplay of personal and transpersonal energies reveals a powerful and mystical dimension to this chakra, its issues and functioning. The fifth chakra governs the transcendent experience of creating. True creativity requires an opening to something greater than self. This premise is easy to understand if we think about inspired, masterful painters, sculptors, or spiritual visionaries. However, creativity also applies to creation of one's self and one's life. Giving expression to oneself is an act of creation. To give full, meaningful expression to oneself, one must surrender self-consciousness, self-judgment, and self-denial and *allow* what is inside self – emotions, ideas, desires, vision, needs, etc. – to come forth.

Your throat chakra acts as the on-off switch for your creative energy, and the control for the switch belongs to you alone. The on-off positions reflect your internal permission for *or* restriction of self-expression, respectively. They also reflect your willingness to permit *or* your desire to restrict the self-expression of others. The key word for the *on* position is *allowing* – a willingness and ability to let self, another, or a situation *be*. The key word for the *off* position is *negating* – an unwillingness and inability to allow self, another, or situation *to be*. Negating may take the form of force, coercion, judgment, restriction of expression, or control. When the switch is in the *on* position, you receive electrical charge, the life force to exist and to be. When the switch is in the *off* position, you withhold life force energy from yourself and a part of you is not allowed to be.

You can recognize if your fifth chakra switch is *on* or *off* by feeling your throat. *Is your throat open and relaxed, or is it tense, tight or closed?* (If you find it difficult to recognize the feeling in your throat, notice how your jaw and neck feel.) If you feel open and relaxed, your throat is *on*. If you feel tight or closed, your throat is *off*. You can also recognize on-off positions by your own inner attitudes of acceptance, curiosity, and interest *or* judgment, criticism, and rejection. **Every time you allow self, someone, or something to** *be*, **creative potential exists. Every time you negate self, someone, or something, creative potential is lost.**

If you determine that your throat chakra is in the off position, you can train yourself to turn it to *on*. To turn it on, you should first identify who and what you are attempting to negate, force, or restrict. *Are you refusing to feel your own anger, grief, or even fatigue? Are you rejecting a decision or a need of your sister, child, or partner?* If you do not recognize who or what you are trying to suppress, you may still proceed with the energetic focus described below.

If you are negating or suppressing your own feelings, place a pillow over your solar plexus and begin to relax your stomach. Hold the pillow against your stomach until this area relaxes and softens. Then gently focus in your heart chakra and after a few moments begin to consciously relax and open your throat. As energy begins to move, your emotions will rise to the surface. As you become conscious of what you are feeling, *listen*. Listening is an act of receptivity that will allow your emotions to live and evolve. *Feel the emotion*. If you wish to cry, *cry*. If you wish to speak the message of the emotions aloud, *speak*. Continue to use this method of relaxing and listening on a daily basis or until the issues at hand feel healed and integrated.

If you feel unable or unwilling to accept the decision, expression, or a need of another person, you can again use the pillow method of relaxing your stomach followed by focusing in your heart. As energy begins to move in your body, listen to your feelings. You will hear your concerns, your fears, and/or your beliefs about the situation or other person. As your receptivity to your feelings and thoughts increases, your negative attachment will decrease and you will gain energy.

Communicating your concerns, fears, and beliefs to the person involved will support the energetic openness of your throat chakra. You may choose to speak in person or write a letter. If you feel that he or she would not be receptive to you, you can communicate psychically by simply saying the words aloud while seeing yourself in his or her presence.

As you continue to practice connecting with yourself and receptively listening, your body and energy will bring you to a higher level of emotional integrity. And, you will find that

space. Through this discipline a healer deepens her or his ability to *see* and influence positive change.

I have always included this exercise as part of classes and trainings for two reasons. First, seeing is a necessary and valuable spiritual faculty. Second, the ability to contribute to the healing of another or oneself springs from the basic human desire *to help*. There are many times in life when healing resources are needed or when no solution to a problem seems clear. Prayer is one of the most positive, productive ways to contribute to and influence these situations.

Common Benefits and Applications: The Prayer Exercise can effectively help you or others when any form of healing is required. You can use this exercise as a complement to therapy and emotional process work, as well as to medical treatments and procedures. In these cases, the prayer focus promotes inner calm and self-awareness in the prayer recipient, thus contributing to the success of the other healing methods employed.

When using The Prayer Exercise for self-healing, you may have found it surprising to bring a part of yourself in front of you. Within certain healing modalities, this is a common and useful practice. Each of us has an overall identity and psyche. However, individual personas or selves also exist in us and can hold a great deal of energy. These parts of self are connected to a particular time period or occurrence. For example, if you were three years old when your father died, your three-year-old self would be part of that specific event and circumstance. A part of you and your energy, therefore, would reside in this self and would remain overly attached to that event until the experience was fully resolved.

When a part of you is unresolved emotionally, the specific emotions held by that part – fear, grief, sense of abandonment, etc. – continue to live within you and surface when this self is triggered. An unresolved self will affect your inner sense of wholeness and well-being because of the vulnerability and/or trauma she or he carries. The Prayer Exercise offers a way to directly and intimately reconnect with and heal these parts.

The Prayer Exercise may be useful when therapy has failed to work, or when, for some reason, it is not available. This exercise will help you gain awareness of deep or camouflaged aspects of your own emotions and behaviors. Attention given to a specific part of self will help you *digest and evolve* your past pain, isolation, reactions, and misunderstandings. As this psychic evolution progresses, you will experience energetic, emotional, and/or psychological benefits.

Once you gain practice with the focusing methods offered in The Prayer Exercise, try challenging yourself to use this form of prayer work anytime you experience difficulty with someone. However, in these cases rather than actively creating an intention, allow yourself to simply *see*. Through heart vision, you will be able to see beneath the surface of the situation to the deeper causal levels. You will then be able to approach the person and situation in a more informed and compassionate way.

Common Challenges: The greatest challenge for students practicing this exercise has been maintaining receptivity and openness. The reasons for this vary from person to person. Some individuals are very strong-willed; they move through life taking control of themselves and situations. Being receptive is not familiar or comfortable. To release control and *allow something to occur* is foreign. Continued practice with this exercise, especially while using the mudra for detachment, has helped students learn how to be receptive.

Some students have difficulty with this exercise because they have built up defenses in their hearts and have strong inclinations to turn away from intimacy, from hurt, or from anything that they deem unpleasant. Seeing *is* intimate and causes one to feel. Seeing develops courage, and feeling allows the pain to evolve.

If you find that staying present in your heart challenges you, make a commitment to *see* and *feel* in small increments. Practice The Prayer Exercise with yourself, holding your focus for as long as you can remain receptive (this might be as little as three minutes at a time), then commit to return to this focus the following day. Over time, you will become more comfortable with the experience. It may also be helpful for you to connect with your specific personas who are holding defenses. Although this can be a challenge, you will be able to bring inner resolution and transformation by being present and patient.

When working with a part of yourself who is very hurt or defensive, you may experience this self turning away from you during The Prayer Exercise. His or her turning away reveals much. Internally, this part of you has felt isolated for a considerable period of time, does not trust others, and likely does not trust you.

As you read this, you may find the idea of a part of yourself not trusting you far-fetched or ridiculous. However, in terms of energetic and spiritual healing, it is common. We often negate who we are and disown parts of ourselves. We do it through judgment, denial, and defenses that block our true emotions. Once we negate a part of self, a dilution of spirit and loss of self occur.

When you practice The Prayer Exercise, you open the possibility of reconnecting with parts of self *who have been abandoned and isolated.* This reconnection can be a challenge, especially if you cannot open and stabilize your heart chakra. If you experience this, using the mudra for detachment will help you maintain your focus. I also recommend that you do some journal work or inner processing to discover the judgments or fears that you carry about this part of yourself. Once you discover what they are, forgive yourself for harboring them. Then proceed with The Prayer Exercise, working slowly over several sittings. Over time, you will see progress and you will *feel* it.

Energetic Influence: The Prayer Exercise brings an opening and a deepening to the heart chakra that allow unconditional acceptance and love to be more readily available. It also develops an inner stability that will help you utilize your emotional and mental energy more effectively. Both of these improvements will support your energy system by increasing your capacity to receive and retain energy.

Opening the Physical Channel

Course Purpose: Opening the Physical Channel is an essential energetic practice. This exercise focuses on the core of the body and, thus, awakens the center points of all the major chakras. Energetically all chakras are stimulated and refreshed. The emphasis on ascending energy further influences you by lifting the center of your body and energetically connecting the first and seventh chakras. When these two centers are simultaneously awakened and resonant, body-centered meditation occurs.

Whenever and wherever you can practice the correct postural alignment and openness, you will feel this natural, gentle meditation begin. As you become more accomplished at opening your physical channel, you will begin to rely on your body as an energetic instrument, trusting it as the gateway to – and the ground for – spiritual experience.

Practitioners and clinicians, who may need the focus of a meditative state during a session but do not wish to divert their attention from their client, can use this practice with their eyes open.

Common Benefits and Applications: This exercise remedies most types of fatigue. Maintaining openness and healthy ascending and descending flows allows the body to receive a greater amount of life force energy. One's state of mind and sense of well-being are improved. Through the physical channel glandular centers also become energized as the center of the chakras awaken.

You may find it helpful and fun to practice this exercise whenever you are walking or hiking, because opening the physical channel gives buoyancy to the body. When using this application simply open the soles of your feet, relax your knees, and walk. When you experience buoyancy or *uplift* in your body, you will know you are receiving ascending energy. Normally you do not need to attend to descending balance. If you do want to check it, however, you can wait until you have completed your exercising and then state your intention that ascending and descending energies balance. You can use this application of the exercise to reduce muscle pain when backpacking, hiking or walking for great distances, or for easing chronic back, knee, or joint tension.

Opening the Physical Channel also supports a fuller sexual experience in which sexual and spiritual energies are well integrated. Increased flow of energy through the chakra system, auric field, and physical channel facilitates sexual union on both personal and transcendent levels. (You may wish to review this information in the Context.)

To practice this application, I would recommend that you and your partner both use the sitting position of this exercise for ten to fifteen minutes before making love. Spend the latter part of this time looking into each other's eyes (while still holding your physical channel focus). Then release your focus as you normally would in meditation practice *or* simply follow your own desires and instincts.

Intentionally opening your physical channel can assist you in transforming your consciousness, because the ascending energy helps to release both energetic and physical blocks. **When the body holds blockages, the mind harbors defenses, and vice versa.** When the body releases stress, the mind experiences greater harmony. Spontaneously, inner harmony will begin to express itself through your thoughts, words, and actions, improving and blessing your relationships with self, others, and the Earth. I consider an open physical channel foundational to physical-spiritual balance and to the practice of nonviolence.

Common Challenges: Students often feel challenged by the physical alignment part of the exercise. Chronic poor posture and back or knee problems bring certain complications to finding proper positioning. However, *without fail,* every student successfully opens the physical channel simply by making small, often subtle adjustments to her or his posture. Even students with curvature of the spine have been able to open their physical channel and feel the energy lifting them upwards. The key to this exercise is to remember that your physical channel exists as part of your *energetic instrument.* In this regard, it knows itself, and on some level, you already know your physical channel. Trust this. If, after several practices, you discover the sitting position works better for you than the standing one, or vice versa, solely practice that one. In the weeks and months that follow, you can try all positions again and will likely enjoy greater comfort and success with each.

Occasionally, students have been challenged by the openness they feel when practicing this exercise. They describe feeling more emotionally and energetically exposed to the world and other people. This feeling usually results from the spontaneous release of defenses and remains only until you have adapted to being more open. If you find that you still feel uncomfortable after a couple of weeks, you may want to work with a healing practitioner or utilize The Prayer Exercise to discover and resolve the deeper level of your experience.

Energetic Influence: Opening the Physical Channel strengthens the capacity of your body to conduct vital energy by allowing the body to optimally fulfill one of its key energetic functions – receiving ascending energy. The energy gain here is substantial, yet consistently absorbs well. This exercise increases core physical stability and brings confidence to all other meditation practice.

Reference Point Meditation

Course Purpose: The Reference Point Meditation introduces you to the soul center within your heart chakra. I chose the name *reference point* because it is in the soul center where true discernment and knowing abides. All concerns, decisions, and choices can be brought to this physical-energetic center to be processed. Processing here is integrative and spiritually empowering. Perspective and truth gained in the reference point reflect the inherent intelligence of your soul.

This meditation requires a refined and subtle focus as you concentrate and become aware of the energy flow within and around you. This awareness initiates a gentle centering process while creating a powerful stillness. The reference point or soul center is the still point within you. It is the place where all chaos ceases.

Common Benefits and Applications: The Reference Point Meditation offers a pure, deep energetic experience that gently and deeply nourishes the nervous system. You may use this meditation as a nervous system detoxifier, as it facilitates inner peace and reconnection. Using the meditation on a regular basis will also strengthen your connection with your heart chakra and help you cultivate compassion and integrate heart vision into your life.

You will find that connecting to your reference point develops a general receptivity to life and promotes emotional and mental neutrality. The combination of receptivity and neutrality fosters clear spiritual vision and knowing – the ability to recognize *what is*, as opposed to what you interpret or project. As you practice and develop these abilities, you will find that your mental stress is profoundly reduced and your intuitive and instinctual abilities increase.

Common Challenges: The challenge students most often experience with the Reference Point Meditation rests in learning how to hold a dual focus during the meditation – centering in your deep heart while maintaining awareness of energy circulation. If you find that you have difficulty with your focus, first reinforce your connection in your reference point. Deepening this connection will improve your overall concentration. Then remember that you need only be aware of the circulation of energy; you *do not* need to make the energy circulate.

If during any given practice of this meditation, you cannot achieve dual focus – rely solely on your connection to your reference point. This singular focus will successfully prepare you for the next practice.

Energetic Influence: This meditation gives you an opportunity to exercise and strengthen your energy system and connect with your deep heart. The energy gain experienced in the Reference Point Meditation automatically integrates through the energy circulation within and around you.

Soul Force Meditation

Course Purpose: Every person has a soul, a unique, individual intelligence of specific energetic qualities, that encompasses the combined energy of **will,** volition of one's spirit; **context,** life experiences, orientation, and karma; and **resources,** knowledge, values, abilities, and spiritual alliances.

The soul's vital energy is called *soul force.* This vital energy emanates through and from the deep heart chakra and may be conducted through the body via the energy system that serves as both the receiver and transmitter of this energy. Transmitting or channeling your soul force gives your soul *energetic presence* in your life and attunes your body to the soul's frequency.

Channeling soul force constitutes a personal, initiatory step in spiritual growth. As you have proceeded through the meditation practices, you have developed and strengthened your energy system. In doing so, you have also learned to care for and protect your own energy. Now, you are able to receive your soul force and be a more conscious guardian of it *and* a container for it.

Common Benefits and Applications: Each person values the Soul Force Meditation according to his or her own sensibilities and life experience. My appreciation for it comes from years sharing in the growth processes of students. I have heard many people struggle with their concept of God and doubt their own spiritual worthiness. I have watched others forcefully strive toward enlightenment and give away their own power to teachers or gurus. I have seen some teachers and gurus encourage this. I value this soul force practice because it brings the soul energy to the body and promotes a *personal experience* of spiritual identity and self-recognition. These realizations are essential to selfhood, creating an internal foundation upon which spiritual potential can be gracefully actualized.

The Soul Force Meditation, like the Reference Point Meditation, offers calm, energetic nourishment that strengthens the nervous system. It also enhances your physical well-being by providing a gentle expansion and clearing within the energy system. Regular use of this meditation supports the heart chakra as well as the thymus chakra and will, therefore, clarify the issues and life activities governed by both.

Your soul force offers a practical compass for everyday life. It is an incredible resource that will support you when you are faced with a challenging decision-making process or when you wish to awaken your own creativity and vision. I recommend connecting with your soul force when you are emotionally drained or depressed. In these situations, the energetic strength and intelligence of your own soul will restore balance and help you regain perspective.

Common Challenges: Soul force comes through the body as a single frequency, which can feel quite subtle. If your soul force energy is extraordinarily light, of a very high vibratory rate, you may find it challenging to perceive – especially if you expect an energetic experience similar to Opening the Physical Channel or the Heart and Crown Meditation.

Differing from the preceding practices in the series, this last meditation accesses purely transcendent energy. You likely have never – or rarely – experienced energy of this quality before. Therefore, you will have to remain present and alert to recognize it. Sometimes the first identifiable sign of your soul force is an opening of the space around you or within you. This *spaciousness* translates into many levels of internal experience, such as peace, lucid awareness, connection to infinite reality, etc., which you will begin to notice as you stay with your focus.

Soul force often feels physically and energetically illuminating, especially in your thymus and throat chakras, both of which are naturally resonant with higher frequency energy. Another delightful sign of soul force energy is a gentle, involuntary smile that – through the radiance of your *being* – lights your face. You do not have to see this light to know it is there, *you will feel it*. The key to recognizing these signs and perceiving the frequency of your soul force is in-the-moment sensory awareness, which comes from keeping still and deep in your reference point.

A common challenge that arises with the Soul Force Meditation is that students do not trust that their soul force will come through when called upon. Usually in these cases the channeling begins and then abruptly stops, because the person begins to question it. The doubt, as well as poor concentration, draws the person from his or her deep heart.

If you experience this challenge, focus on staying *physically deep* in the reference point. As you channel your soul force energy, you can occasionally remind yourself to focus deeper in your reference point. To further encourage yourself, consider the image of inserting a plug into a socket. When your concentration slips from deep heart to shallow heart, the flow of your soul force energy will diminish – *your plug has slipped out of the socket*. To re-focus, push back into your deep heart and the current of your soul force will increase.

Students who are emotionally reserved or physically inactive are sometimes challenged by the sensation of soul force energy in their bodies. As with Opening the Physical Channel, the Soul Force Meditation awakens the body and the glandular centers. This can *turn the body on* and you may even feel a sexual surge. This feeling is natural, however, and generally balances out as the meditation progresses. If you feel uncomfortable with this meditation, I recommend that you first practice transmitting soul force into your body only. Or, you may wish to let your soul force resonate in your heart chakra only. Practicing either modified method will allow you to channel less energy. When you feel ready to progress to a fuller energetic experience, let your soul force flow through your hands and into the room. Channeling using your hands will help you become more familiar with the energetic qualities of your soul force.

You should know that when channeling soul force into the room, there is no threat of wasting your energy. Soul force is abundant; its presence in a room will nourish you. It will not deplete you in any way. You can equate transmitting into the room with practicing the Reference Point Meditation. Your soul force energy will circulate back to you in a natural way.

As has been mentioned earlier, it is not appropriate to channel your soul force to *or* for other people past the initial learning and feedback stage (if you are working in a group). If you channel or resonate your soul force near someone who is not consciously aware of what is happening, he or she may inflow your energy in some way. The person receiving your soul energy will then interpret the experience according to his or her own needs and orientation. This individual might equate the feeling of your soul force with love, sexual attraction, needed nurturing, etc. In quite an innocent way, this can lead to confusion or major complications in relationships. To avoid this potential problem, remember that, like your aura, *your soul force is only for you.*

Energetic Influence: The Soul Force Meditation can be considered a *conversion point* to greater energetic and spiritual volume. Your soul force infuses you with the frequency that is unique to you. It expands the quantity and quality of your energy in perfect resonance with who you are. Your soul energy also nourishes your body and nervous system in the most natural and comforting way. The greater influence of this practice, however, exists within your consciousness, as you enjoy more receptivity to your own will and soul directives.

Epilogue

THE SOUL FORCE MEDITATION BEGINS YOUR TRANSITION from the course structure to a self-directed practice. This new cycle can be both exhilarating and isolating, and your success with it depends largely on your ability to make a leap – in focus, in self-love, and in commitment. To support you in this process the Epilogue presents six simple guidelines for making the energetic practices an integrated part of your life. It also offers ways to navigate life changes and identify and reset goals. The Epilogue closes with words of encouragement and direction to help you connect with the Earth and in turn be more deeply guided by her.

How to Continue Your Energetic Practices

The nine exercises in this book may now blur together in your mind. This is natural. At a certain stage of your process, method becomes secondary and your energetic practice becomes purely about your in-the-moment experience. However, now as you transition out of the course structure, the individual exercises and their specific steps again become relevant. These varied self-care tools will help you expand the energetic foundation you have just built and create a personal practice that works for you.

Begin with Soul Force

Upon your completion of the course work, I recommend that you continue to practice the Soul Force Meditation at least three times a week for approximately two weeks. This meditation can be simplified by resonating your soul force in your heart chakra only. Or, you can let your soul force fill your entire body and auric field rather than transmitting it into a room. These two weeks of practice will help you recognize your soul's signature vibration and qualities. Energetically, you are learning to attune to the greater part of you and accept its restorative influence in your daily life.

No Pleasure, No Gain

During or immediately following the two weeks of practicing soul force, I suggest that you review your journal and the Energetic Practices section of the book. Beyond the techniques themselves, remember how each practice affected you – how each balanced, strengthened, or awakened you. Creating an ongoing energetic practice *that works for you* needs to start with the exercises that you love. These are the practices that speak to you in an essential way. They soothe, energize, or nourish something in you that needs attending to. Listen to them and listen to what you love.

Check in with Yourself

The next step in creating your practice is to accept that checking in with yourself energetically, on a daily basis, is just as important as taking in food and water. Set the intention to check in with yourself at least once a day. You can do this in the morning or before you go to bed in the evening. You can check in upon your return from work or in the car before you leave work. It will not matter if you check your heart chakra, your aura, your physical channel, or how much energy you expend on a particular day. Making this contact strengthens your connection and commitment to self. Checking in does not require doing an exercise. Checking in simply helps you *listen*. It is a way to demonstrate self-love.

Put Practice on Your Calendar

Taking responsibility for your time and how you use it is an important energy exercise. Rushing, overdoing, and running late will drain your energy. Crowding the day with so much that you have no time for yourself depletes you and misuses your energy. Supporting yourself energetically means that you manage time responsibly in order to attend to what is important **at a pace that is energetically healthy.**

With this in mind, consider energetic practice as a means of restoring your natural equilibrium and balancing your pace. Practice need only take 10-20 minutes three times per week. Or you may prefer to spend time every day. *This is entirely up to you.* Consider your monthly and weekly schedules. Notice if there is a consistent time of day available for you and your practice. If you do not have time every day, *accept* that. If you have no consistent time week to week, *accept* that and pencil in an irregular schedule of appointments with yourself.

These personal practice times are as important to your life as all the other engagements you have planned. In fact, they form the foundation for all the others. When you meet with yourself, work with your favorite energetic exercise or work with one that would best serve your present needs. Your practice will then become the energetic support structure of your life. **If you miss a practice day with yourself, do not worry.** Place your hands over your heart for five minutes and look forward to your next date with yourself.

Use What You Know in Times of Stress

Challenge yourself to use the practices for neutralizing stress. When you are struggling with making an important decision or recovering from a long day at work – **stop.** *Does your third chakra hurt? Are you losing energy in a specific direction? Is your first chakra closed down? Are you tired?* **Before you take an aspirin, drink a cup of coffee, or eat a brownie:** put your hands over your heart, open the chakras at the bottom of your feet, place a seal around your auric field, or practice the Inflow Exercise. Spontaneous use of the energetic practices will strengthen you three-fold and leave you refreshed in mind and body.

You Are Your Own Guardian

Creating an energetic practice that supports you depends on much more than focus and time. It depends on self-love, self-interest, and the wisdom to recognize that **you are the one who is responsible for taking care of yourself. You are the first-responder.** You are the first one who feels your distress, the first one who can address it, and the first one who can ask for help when needed. Acting from this knowledge will support you in using the energetic practices, *and* using the energetic practices will strengthen your ability to respond to yourself in a loving, committed way.

Life Adjustments and Further Integration

The developmental practices of this course have strengthened your energy system and expanded its capacity to receive, conduct, transmit, and retain energy. This improvement in energetic function can influence many levels of your experience.

The first influence you notice is immediate and energetic. For example, the moment you place a seal around your aura or focus in your deep heart, you are no longer diffuse or no longer shallow-hearted. Diffuseness and shallowness are energetic behaviors as much as they are emotional and psychological ones. You can feel immediate changes in energetic behavior in the body and energy system. Your breathing may deepen, your spine straighten, and/or your heart chakra open. These responses are often accompanied by an increased sense of well-being, self-awareness, and peace.

As you incorporate new energetic behaviors, you begin to adjust attitudes and actions. *You probably have noticed this already*. If you have functioned with a diffuse aura for many years, a sealed one can give you a sense of healthy detachment or containment, or it can give you the life-altering ability to finally say "no." You will also feel more self-interested and motivated to attend to what you like to do.

If you have functioned with a shallow heart, being in your deep heart will result in less self-criticism, a more consistent connection with your own truth, and/or an increased capacity for forgiveness. You may find that you feel calmer about things or people that once irritated you. You may experience less anger or less fear.

As you can imagine – or as you have already experienced – transformation in attitude and behavior rapidly affects how you interact with other people. This level of change can be both healing and challenging as it opens new territory in your intimate, casual, and professional relationships. You may be pleasantly surprised, frustrated, or even saddened by what you discover.

Some people in your life will welcome the changes within you and deepen their connection with you. Others may feel threatened and want you to behave in a way that is familiar. Some people may totally resist your changes. They might openly challenge you and/or distance themselves. If you can step back and look through your heart, you will most often discover that relationships that truly give you energy remain intact and strengthen, and those that fail to nourish you or that drain you, fall away.

When you find that you want or need to actively facilitate adjustments in relationships, you must truthfully represent yourself and allow others to do the same. If doing this is a new experience for you, take time to listen internally to what you authentically feel. Clarifying what you want, prefer, or need in your own mind first, then sharing it, develops invaluable communication skills. Encouraging other people to follow suit is essential. When each person brings his or her truth forward, transformation happens. Intimacy and respect increase and personal differences and insecurities become secondary.

As you continue your integration process, you will benefit from reviewing and re-evaluating your lifestyle, personal goals, and perhaps even your career. The intention here is not to force change upon areas that are working, but rather to make appropriate changes in areas that are failing to nourish you or are draining you. This personal assessment process does not have to be done in a linear or analytical way. It can be done in a spontaneous, nurturing fashion by simply listening to and recording your needs, dreams, and fantasies. In each of these resides an essential part of you.

Creativity is connected with the *allowing will* and the soul. Exploring your needs, wants, fantasies, and dreams with interest and curiosity will help you understand their messages. You may discover that you want to change your diet or buy a new wardrobe. You may realize that you want to establish a five-year plan to accommodate further education or travel. You may wish to move closer to family or to maintain a greater connection to nature. Whatever life adjustments you set into motion – whether they influence your relationships, your career, or where you take your next vacation – will create greater body-mind-soul cohesiveness and create an outer world that satisfactorily connects with your inner one. Your life is your evolution. Trust yourself.

Embracing the Earth

As you grow in energetic sensitivity, you will naturally extend this awareness beyond yourself and at times experience the field that holds all living things to each other. Penetrate its reality. Eradicate your sense of separation. And, on behalf of all life, embrace the Earth.

Earth is a living entity. She emanates both energy and consciousness. Your energy system, body, soul, and intelligence are linked to the energy field and consciousness of the Earth and are influenced by them. Trust this interconnection *and experiment.* Go to your favorite place in your yard or in your nearest park and lie on the Earth. Close your eyes and notice how energy begins to move in your body. Breathe and let the life force of the Earth balance your energy system – your meridians, chakras, physical channel, and aura. Then try it again the next time you have a headache, a sore throat, or when you are feeling fatigued. You will soon discover that Earth is our ever-present healer.

It is good to fall in love with the Earth, to let yourself discover her unimaginable beauty and celebrate your connection to all living things. You can also let the Earth discover you. The Earth and nature will interact with you through energy. You feel this when you lie on the Earth, stand in a vast, open field, or perch yourself on the edge of an ancient canyon wall. *Pay attention. Earth is speaking with you, opening your heart, and awakening your mind.*

There are specific places on the Earth that will resonate with you and strengthen you more than others. When you find the places that you are deeply connected to, you will know it. You will have greater joy and peace there. Your own thoughts will reveal it; your mind will be clear, calm, and expansive. The unity between your deep heart and your body will be pronounced. Your physical channel will open; your energy system will hum.

The Earth may at times offer you – as it did me – a doorway to a completely transcendent experience. Locations on the Earth that facilitate such events are called *thin places* by some people, *places of the gods* by others, or simply *coordinate points*. A true thin place is an area where Earth vibration closely aligns with the vibration of the nonphysical world creating a point of dimensional interface. These places act as portals between universal or infinite consciousness and beings *and* the Earth and humanity. In populated areas, cathedrals, kivas, or ancient ritual sites often identify these places. In the wilderness, your inner recognition and responsiveness are your only indicators.

To find such a place, I suggest that you travel to areas where your heart and soul feel an affinity – perhaps where much untouched land exists. It is also essential to remember that the right place and your presence there do not always result in an exceptional experience. Relationship based in connection – in your abilities to listen, recognize, respect – is the initiator of any extraordinary contact. Fostering this level of relationship will require receptivity and stillness on your part. Connecting to your reference point and / or your physical channel on a regular basis will strengthen these attributes within you.

If you live in the heart of the city or have spent little time in quiet, natural places, my suggestion to embrace the Earth and nature may seem impractical. However, I believe that it will be well worth your while to venture out of densely populated areas to find a place where Earth energy is not compromised. No matter where you live it is good to go to places where you – your body and consciousness – can fully release accumulated environmental stresses and *just be*.

The Lake

Nearly twenty years after I left the farm and the lake, I returned for a visit. I drove the long journey by myself. I wanted to savor the perceivable stages of leaving populated areas behind – to see and feel the lessening of human design and clutter – and enter the clean landscape of the forests, rivers, lakes, and grasslands. I also needed to make a transition internally, to gradually grow more humble and still in increments.

I was not sure if I would recognize the farm. I was not sure, in mileage, its distance from more obvious landmarks. I saw the lake first. It sparkled *blue* – electric blue in contrast to the autumn-gold grasses. My body recognized the north border of the farm, the rise and fall of the road that I had felt so many times before, and then I saw the poplar grove. It was there in the small curve of the lakeshore. The trees looked thin, empty of leaves due to an early fall storm. The farm seemed larger to me. The old houses we once lived in were gone, completely gone.

As I walked the arc of the hill to the lake, the wind shifted the high, yellow grass at my feet. A transparent pink light filtered through the sky tinting everything in subtle ways. My breaths grew deeper. I felt *home*.

I stayed in the area for almost two weeks. The *hum* of the stillness put me to sleep at night and enveloped me throughout the day. The years that had passed were no longer relevant. The poplar grove, the lake, the hum had remained constant. And, although I had changed, my resonance with them had not. This land and the lake were my teachers. Then and there, I knew how deeply I had taken in their gifts. *I knew.*

Appendix

THIS CLOSING SECTION OF THE BOOK AND COURSE offers follow-up resources for your further exploration of subtle energy, the interplay of energy and health, and deeper physical-spiritual integration. A complete list of the meridian circulation cycles provides you with a means to link time of day to specific organ meridians. An additional three-part exercise serves as an adjunct to your integration work.

I have included a list of key questions commonly asked by clients and class members. I believe my responses will address subjects you too have questioned during this course work. I also include a list of practitioners and organizations I value. The list is personal and select. It reflects my experience, preferences, and temperament. Hopefully it will provide you with a beginning point or add to the network of clinicians and institutions that you currently utilize.

Meridian Cycles

Before reviewing the following list, you may wish to re-read the meridian material in the Context.

Every day a two-hour period of circulatory intensification occurs once within each of the twelve organ meridians. These biorhythmic intervals happen at the same time each day and, thus, can help you identify which organ energies are stressed, depleted, agitated, etc. When you notice a physical, emotional, or energetic disturbance, you can turn to the time chart to locate the meridian that corresponds with the hour of your experience. Repetitive patterns are especially important to recognize.

Once you identify the organ meridian, you can better know how to approach correcting the condition. You might choose to work with a chakra, modify your diet, or enlist the aid of a practitioner of traditional Chinese medicine.

Cycles

1 – 3 A.M. Liver	1 – 3 P.M. Small Intestine
3 – 5 A.M. Lung	3 – 5 P.M. Bladder
5 – 7 A.M. Large Intestine	5 – 7 P.M. Kidney
7 – 9 A.M. Stomach	7 – 9 P.M. Pericardium
9 – 11 A.M. Spleen	9 – 11 P.M. Triple Warmer
11 A.M. – 1 P.M. Heart	11 P.M. – 1 A.M. Gallbladder

Healing Life-Negating Thoughts

Here is a powerful and enlightening three-part exercise to help you release self-negating habits.

In class, we call negative, limiting, or destructive beliefs and thoughts, "leaks," because they misuse and drain vital energy. We call correcting or healing these beliefs/thoughts, "sealing leaks." Learning to seal leaks is essential to maintaining your energetic strength and balance.

Thought, like intention, sets energy into motion. **An intense or forceful thought, whether positive or negative, carries a great deal of energy and velocity.** When a powerful thought is generated it moves forward with energetic strength and creates **with impact.**

Monitoring your thoughts and recognizing the energy they transmit is an important part of energetic and spiritual self-care. Thoughts are a form of personal behavior and, therefore, will nourish, fail to nourish, or drain you. Consider this as you listen to your own thoughts and uncover thought patterns. Learn to focus your thoughts – attitudes, beliefs, and directives – as intentionally as you choose your actions. If you find that your thoughts have great power and velocity, train yourself *to think* with more compassion and neutrality *and* with less righteousness and drama.

As you become experienced at using the following techniques, you will find that you develop an automatic ability to neutralize harmful, defensive, and/or judgmental thinking. Energetically you will become clearer, more open, and more present with *what is*. When you stay alert in this way, judgments and limiting thoughts will no longer have a way to attach to you. Your energy system will retain more energy and your throat chakra will stay *on*.

Exercise I: Thoughts directed toward self

Take a moment to think of a common criticism or judgment you have about yourself.

Now, close your eyes and focus on this judgment.

Notice how your body and energy system feel.

When you have done this, forgive yourself for this thought and let it go. Internally, you may also wish to say, "I love you" or "I see you as you truly are," into your heart chakra.

Questions to answer in your journal:

1. When you held the judgment, did you feel your body contract or tense in some way?
2. Did your chakras clamp shut or certain stress patterns overtake the musculature of your body?

3. Once you forgave yourself, did your body and energy return to normal? *If it did not, repeat the last step again taking more time to be kind to yourself.*

Now, imagine the impact of chronic hurtful thoughts or criticisms on your body and your energy system. **Make a commitment to yourself** to monitor and correct your self-negating thoughts and beliefs.

Exercise II: Thoughts directed toward others

Now, take a moment and focus on a negative thought or judgment that you have about another person.

Close your eyes and notice how your body and energy system feel.

When you have done this, let the thought go, release yourself from the judgment. Forgive yourself for the judgment. Release the other person from the judgment and apologize internally to the other person.

Questions to answer in your journal:

1. When you focused on the judgment, did you feel your body contract or tense in some way?
2. Did your chakras react?
3. Once you forgave yourself and released the judgment, did your body and energy return to normal?
4. Are you surprised to find that negative or limiting thoughts you have about another person also impact your body and energy system?

All thought is energy. Whenever you produce a thought, you emit energy. The energy of any and all thought first influences your energy system, especially your chakras and auric field. The thought either nourishes, fails to nourish, or drains you. Chronic thought patterns create the *psychic oxygen that you breathe*. Repetitive thoughts strongly affect the energy within your aura, which then circulates back into you. Your auric energy, your *oxygen,* can be life-supporting or life-negating.

The energy of your thoughts influences others second. When another person is receptive to your thoughts, he or she may experience physical and energetic responses similar to the ones you feel. Likewise, if you are receptive to another person's thoughts about you, your body and energy system will react accordingly.

Exercise III: Thoughts received from others

Be aware of negative or limiting thoughts that another person has about you. Choose one that you are particularly sensitive about.

Notice how your body feels when you focus on that thought.

Now, take time to notice if you carry a similar belief, judgment, or thought about yourself. *You will likely find a match.*

Now, release the thought of the other person and forgive yourself for the corresponding thought that you harbor about yourself. It is important to make a positive, self-affirming statement in your own heart. Example: "I appreciate who I am. I am willing to be honest and kind with myself. I love myself and I am willing to grow."

If you feel that your self-criticism is founded in some truth, then turn this self-assessment into a positive commitment to learning and/or transforming your behavior. Such dedication to your own well-being *will nourish you.*

Questions to answer in your journal:

1. How did the negative thought from another person influence you emotionally and physically?

2. Did you find a parallel thought within yourself?

3. Were you able to neutralize that thought and release it?

4. Do you feel better now?

Dealing with unfair criticism or the negative thoughts generated by another person can be challenging. It is important to empower yourself in these circumstances. Realize that your own conditioning and critical beliefs about yourself provide an *emotional target* upon which the negative thoughts of others can land. Your targets make you vulnerable to outside criticism and judgment and make it difficult for you to recognize what is true. As you heal negative beliefs about yourself, you will become unreceptive to the harming thoughts of others.

It is always important to remember that judgments and labels are static and stagnating. They create a limited view of any given situation or individual. Truth and self-awareness provide the correct context and will naturally allow for transformation and growth. Experiment with letting go of judgments and labels – and learn to simply state *what is*. In time, you will discover how to use discernment, assessment, and analysis without negative labeling or judging.

Ten Most Frequently Asked Questions

1. Do I have to see or feel energy to do the energetic practices?

No, although your ability to sense energy will come in time. Learning to see and feel energy is a process of reawakening your sensory awareness. Most people have been conditioned to ignore energy. And a percentage of them, unfortunately, have been discouraged from feeling. As a result, the parameters of their perception narrow and a whole range of sensory, emotional, and instinctual awareness is lost.

If you find that you are not feeling energy during the practices, consider this: your sensory awareness has atrophied. I know this is a strong word, but it is an accurate one. Practice is the antidote. Practice will help you strengthen and coordinate your focus, connection, and sensory perception. And at the moment that is right for you, your sensory abilities will begin to expand.

Also, when you complete a practice, remember to write down everything you experienced. Often I find that students see or feel energy, but do not acknowledge it. They have learned to discount their own experience. Do not doubt yourself or fear judgment, simply *feel what you feel, see what you see,* and acknowledge it.

2. Are some people able to work with subtle energy and others aren't? *This question relates to the previous one, yet is different.*

No. Everyone is able to work with subtle energy. However, the *entry point* for truly recognizing energy varies from person to person. One person may connect easily with energy in the heart chakra, another person through the physical channel, another on a hike in the mountains. However, once the *aha moment* happens, energy awareness becomes more accessible.

Working with energy requires receptivity. Being receptive to energy, *or anything,* will confront certain issues. A person who is controlling does not usually find being receptive very appealing. An individual not well grounded in his or her body is not always comfortable feeling energy. Anyone who has been emotionally, sexually, and/or physically abused is understandably less receptive for a period of time. In my experience teaching the practices, however, I have seen every student become more receptive, work with energy, and/or meditate. By practicing different exercises, the ego, the body, and *the gut* become used to energetic experience and its benefits. Sooner or later, a person recognizes the greater sense of "survivability" that energetic awareness and meditation bring.

3. What are the main benefits of meditation?

The benefits of meditation are quite varied depending on the technique used, although there are commonalities. I will address meditation as experienced through the energetic practices.

First, meditation offers a direct way to relax and shift focus from the finite and external world. Internal focus coupled with energy awareness allows us to come into the present moment *and* energetically replenish, restore, and rejuvenate. Additionally, regular meditation practice has an accumulative effect of creating a reservoir of calm and clarity. This reservoir is what I consider one of the great spiritual resources of meditation.

Another incredible benefit of meditation is that it helps to establish a clearer body-mind-spirit connection. This promotes self-knowledge, self-empowerment, and better health.

For some people, however, the greatest benefit of meditation is access to transcendent experience. This path of practice is powerful because it can allow the practitioner interaction with other planes of consciousness and the nonphysical world. When solidly grounded in physical, energetic focus, a practitioner can enjoy sublime peace, gain important insight and information, and receive invaluable spiritual support. This mystic path also develops strong self-referencing skills and a greater ability to connect with and value all life.

4. Why am I not always able to feel my heart chakra and experience my soul force?

The heart chakra governs many life issues, one of which is acceptance of self and others. During the day-to-day activities of life, you can subtly or *not so* subtly deny love and compassion. This can happen through discounting or disconnecting from self or others. You might override your fatigue or not listen to a friend who is trying to speak with you. What may seem like a small incident can have a strong impact. If these behaviors intensify or if you are an energetically sensitive person, your heart chakra will likely close or congest, leaving access to the reference point compromised.

If your heart chakra closes easily or frequently, you might find it helpful to connect with your heart on a daily basis, using the Self-Nurturing Meditation or Hands Over Heart. If your heart closes because of a chronic pattern of denial or negation of self, be patient and work on the underlying emotional cause. You should also continue to energetically connect with your heart chakra on a regular basis.

5. I am very busy and do not practice enough, how can I correct this?

If you consistently cannot find time for practice, you need to question your connection with yourself. You need to explore what keeps you from yourself. There may be old wounds or conditioning that negate your needs or self-respect. You may also want to question whether you are avoiding internal information about yourself. Limiting self-connection can keep certain emotions and truths submerged.

On a lighter note, if you occasionally forget about your practice time, do not concern yourself. Be spontaneous. When you have a moment, *do a practice*. Spontaneity can make your overall practice better fit your lifestyle and life rhythms.

6. Can children learn these practices?

Yes, but keep in mind that children are less *psychically cluttered* than most adults, which means they are more facile in their consciousness. Some of the practices are more complex in method than children need. However, the core purpose of each practice can be conveyed to children, and, with a little direction, they can run with it. For instance, the Heart and Crown Meditation is too much, although looking through the eyes of the heart would be great. I do not feel the entire self-care sequence is appropriate. I suggest that you simply follow the interest and practical needs of the child. And, of course, if the child *does not get it* or *want to do it*, never push.

7. How do I speak about the practices with friends and family who are not familiar with subtle energy and energetic self-care?

You can start with words or concepts that are recognizable. Meditation or holistic healing may be familiar terms. It also helps to remember that knowledge of energy is present within every person on some level – after all, we are all energetic beings. When I speak with people about healing or energy, I know and *feel* that our common nature aids in the discussion. Consider this bond when speaking with others.

I suggest that you take time to write your own thoughts about the practices and energy. If what you want to say is clear to you, others are more likely to understand.

8. How do I continue to learn about energy?

First take time to ground your connection to the nine practices in this book. These practices are not categorized as beginning or advanced in level. They simply address the key functions of your energy system, utilize a greater range of your consciousness, and nourish your physical-spiritual health. These needs for self-care are constant and, therefore, the practice series can remain a part of your life over many, many years.

Continued use of the practices will ensure that you become solidly, energetically connected with yourself. The healing aspects of the practices will deepen your transformational process and clear poor energetic habits and conditioning. As you develop more facility with energy, you will become what I call *spiritually buoyant*. That is a state of mind and energy that comes when you identify with the greater, infinite part of yourself and are able to support your internal growth with compassion, wisdom, and curiosity.

Once this level of inner connectedness occurs, you will be well grounded in body-mind-soul self-knowledge, which is an important prerequisite for meaningful exploration of energy. I suggest that you then listen to your body and heart to hear your next step. You will likely know exactly what you want to learn or experience. The resource list that follows may give you some ideas for complementary work.

9. Which of the nine exercises will mostly directly help me with physical health?

The energy system is the ground from which health springs. Physical conditions and illnesses begin as energetic-consciousness conditions – life-negating beliefs, undigested emotions, depleted energy, etc. Sometimes these stresses do not manifest in the body. Sometimes we have karmic grace periods with them; other times we do not. Listening to your energy system on a regular basis will help you know your body and, therefore, protect your overall well-being. Once something is physically manifested, working with your energy system aids in partially or totally redirecting the condition.

Each practice has an effect on your health because each strengthens the energy system. However, if you have a specific condition or illness that you are currently dealing with, try to understand it in terms of energy. For instance, is your condition a stagnation of energy? Or, does it reflect a weakening of energy? Is it a form of toxicity or a form of self-attack? If you can discern the energetic quality of your condition or illness, you can match it up with a practice that most directly addresses and corrects it.

It is always helpful to notice how your body feels when you use a specific practice. This will give you very grounded information about how the exercise affects you physically. The chakras have a dynamic influence on the body. Chakra work, therefore, will open up the dialogue between you and your body, which can quickly result in improved health by increasing the chakra's ability to receive, transmit, and retain energy. Always refer to the chakra nearest to the location of your physical stress or illness for it will be linked to the causal factor of your health challenge.

The physical channel is also a powerful healing tool because it opens a total flow of energy and transports stress, thought patterns, and defenses from form to formlessness. It will quickly relieve joint pain, back pain, and certain headaches. Opening the Physical Channel also eases sciatica. Personally I find that the Soul Force Meditation improves my physical energy, as does Clearing and Sealing the Auric Field. The Reference Point Meditation will re-gather energy and restore balance – which is quite helpful if you are stressed and racing on adrenaline.

With all health concerns, it is critical that you recognize when professional help is needed and seek proper care. **It is also important to validate your self-knowledge** and the healing power of energetic self-care. If you already work with *or* can find a health practitioner who has an integrative approach, you will be able to bring your insights and practices to him or her.

10. Do we all have spirit guides? And if so, how do I contact them?

In my experience, most people have some relationship with beings who occupy the nonphysical or spirit world. However, most people are not aware of these relationships.

I honestly do not know any direct, sure-fire way to contact a guide. I feel it is always productive to cultivate stillness and calm. In deeper states of meditation or focus, you may experience lucid moments of contact. However, do not create grand expectations of what meeting with these beings should be. In my experience, connection and communication with other-dimensional folks is subtle, though sometimes very emotional and sometimes funny. Their words often enter at the sixth chakra or come as thoughts that *breeze through the mind.*

In some cultures the spirit world is accepted as a constant, expected, and real part of life. And, therefore, it is absurd to imagine that we are ever alone. That being said, the subject of guides is a very personal one. If you believe in guides and other dimensional companions, then listen for them. And if you are closed to the possibility, do not concern yourself with the subject at all.

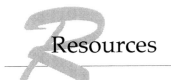

Resources

Elizabeth Frediani conducts individual and group classes and mentorship programs. She maintains a private healing practice in Pennsylvania and Washington State. To read more about her work or to contact her, go to www.elizabethfrediani.com or email Elizabeth@elizabethfrediani.com.

Dr. Robert Ullman and
Dr. Judyth Reichenberg-Ullman
Northwest Center of Homeopathy
131 Third Ave. N
Edmonds, WA 98020
(425) 774-5599

Robert Jangaard, Naturopathic Physician
Jangaard Clinic
1657 E. Layton Rd.
Freeland, WA 98249
(360) 331-6470

Sandra Ingerman
P.O. Box 4757
Santa Fe, NM 87502
www.sandraingerman.com

Bastyr Center for Natural Health
3670 Stone Way N
Seattle, WA 98103
(206) 834-4100

Jin Shin Jyutsu Inc.
8719 E. San Alberto Dr.
Scottsdale, AZ 85258
(480) 998-9331

Shoshana Sadow,
M. Ac., L.Ac. Dipl.Ac.
Centro Integral de Salud
Oaxaca, Mexico
011-52-951-516-0906

Sunny Chu, Herbal Doctor
Sunny's Herbs
Shoreline, WA
(206) 363-2028

Dr. Chen
Sun Acupuncture
7007 E. Hampton Ave.
Denver, CO   80224
(303) 756-1166

ISSSEEM – The International Society for the Study of Subtle
Energies and Energy Medicine
11005 Ralston Rd., Suite 210
Arvada, CO 80004
www.issseem.org

American Holistic Nurses Association
323 N. San Francisco
Suite 201
Flagstaff, AZ 86001
www.ahna.org

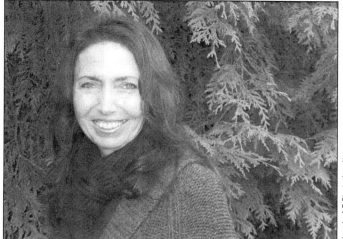

Photo by A. T. Birmingham-Young

About the Author

Elizabeth Frediani's work with subtle energy healing practices began in 1972 and was an integral part of her life in the North American wilderness of British Columbia. After ten years of study to fully understand her ability to see and feel energy, she created a whole system of energy-centered meditation practices and healing techniques, which include the Psychic Cord Release Process,[SM] the Past Life Resolution Process,[SM] and the material presented in this book. In 1984 she founded the Transformational Healing Institute in Boulder, Colorado and directed the school for seven years.

Elizabeth currently works in private practice, teaches, and facilitates group and individual mentorship programs in Pennsylvania and in Washington State. Her recent teaching projects include The Practice of Peace: Nonviolence for Personal and Social Transformation[SM] and trainings for Chakra Clearing with Applied Integration.[SM]

Where Body Meets Soul is Elizabeth's first book. It explores the profound interrelationship between subtle energy and health, consciousness, and spirituality.

Qualified Instructors

The varied courses developed and taught by Elizabeth Frediani, which include The Soul Force Series: Energetic Meditation and Self-Care Practices,[SM] The Practice of Peace: Nonviolence for Personal and Social Transformation,[SM] and Will, Power, Creativity, and Knowing: Reuniting with the Source,[SM] offer instruction to aid individuals in their own self-healing and personal development. Participating in these classes does not qualify or authorize an individual to teach the material.

As Elizabeth continues working with her mentorship groups, prospective teachers are being trained who exemplify integrity, proficiency, and professional, as well as personal, commitment in specific subjects and fields of practice.

In order to preserve continuity in training for the Psychic Cord Release Process,[SM] first named Psychic Cord Work in 1983, and the Past Life Resolution Process,[SM] Elizabeth remains the sole authorized teacher of these practices.

If you have any questions about this statement or would like further information on a related topic, please email Elizabeth@ elizabethfrediani.com.

— Notes —

CPSIA information can be obtained at www.ICGtesting.com
Printed in the USA
BVOW06s1550120913

330939BV00003B/50/P